KIM VOPNI
THE VAGINA COACH

Your Pelvic Floor

A Practical Guide to Solving Your Most Intimate Problems

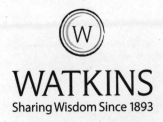

WATKINS
Sharing Wisdom Since 1893

This edition published in the UK and Ireland 2021 by
Watkins, an imprint of Watkins Media Limited
Unit 11, Shepperton House
89-93 Shepperton Road
London
N1 3DF

enquiries@watkinspublishing.com

3 5 7 9 10 8 6 4 2

Designed and typeset by Lapiz

Printed and bound in the United Kingdom by TJ Books Ltd.

A CIP record for this book is available from the British Library

ISBN: 978-1-78678-486-5 (Paperback)
ISBN: 978-1-78678-487-2 (eBook)

www.watkinspublishing.com

CONTENTS

ABOUT THE AUTHOR

Kim Vopni is a self-professed pelvic health evangelist and is known as "The Vagina Coach". She is a certified fitness professional who became passionate about sharing information on pelvic health after the birth of her first child.

She is a published author, a passionate speaker and women's health educator, as well as a mom to two boys.

Kim is the founder of Pelvienne Wellness Inc – a company offering pelvic health programmes, products and coaching for women in pregnancy, motherhood and menopause. She also cofounded, grew, and sold a company called Bellies Inc where she created the Ab System – a revolutionary birth prep and recovery system for pregnant women. Kim also certifies other fitness and movement professionals to work with women who have core and pelvic floor challenges through her Core Confidence Specialist Certification.

You can find her online at www.vaginacoach.com and on social media @vaginacoach.

ACKNOWLEDGEMENTS

To Anya Hayes and Watkins Publishing – thank you first of all for choosing me and secondly for all of the behind the scenes work that went in to making this book a reality.

To my mom for always answering my questions about your births and body and for telling me the straight facts. Your story and your openness was a huge catalyst for where I am today. You are also the best proofreader I know!

To my dad for moving me (our family) around the world, which has helped me become adaptable, accustomed to change and a lover of travel.

To Tecsana, the makers of the EPI-NO, for creating the amazing product that ultimately started me on this journey.

To my kids for making me a mother.

To Julia Di Paolo and Samantha Montpetit-Huynh for the laughs, the tears and the learning from Bellies Inc.

To my teachers, Diane Lee, Katy Bowman, Julie Wiebe, Jenny Burrell, Michelle Lyons, Antony Lo, Kaisa Tuominen, Tamara Rial and Dr Bruce Crawford for teaching me and giving me the tools to help and inspire others to care about their pelvic health.

To all the pelvic health physios who have supported my work and collaborated with me.

To Myra Robson, co-founder of Pelvicroar and co-creator of the NHS-approved pelvic floor app, Squeezy, for advising on physiotherapy content of the book.

And finally, to my husband, who has talked me off the entrepreneur cliff many times and has been my biggest fan and supporter through it all.

FOREWORD

Every once in a while you meet someone who impresses you with their passion and expertise. It bubbles over not just in joy and enthusiasm but in their absolute commitment to the subject they love. You know when you meet them, even if that subject matter is delicate.

That someone is Kim Vopni, author of *Your Pelvic Floor*. She harnesses all the skills and knowledge she has acquired in her specialist subject to help us change our lives for the better.

Kim cares about your pelvic floor health. Where Kobe Bryant may have focused on the ball and the net, Kim Vopni, the self-titled "Vagina Coach", has focused on that particular part of the female anatomy that is quite possibly the central point of femaleness.

You would think that all those who come equipped with a vagina and a vulva would know how to look after these most intimate parts of the female machinery. That anyone who menstruates knows something about vaginal health, but this knowledge may be the sum total of their vaginal understanding. There is a vast open space of not knowing that can be filled by Kim's knowledge and practical expertise.

I've had the opportunity to participate in Kim's workshops and online programmes. We've also had multiple conversations about wellness, particularly women's health. In one workshop, I learned the Blueberry Visualization technique which you'll find in the book and which, I'm happy to say, has seriously upped my pelvic-floor strengthening game. I also discovered, through Kim's acute eye, that I had a diastasis recti and that I needed to learn how to better engage my abdominal core muscles in order to avoid further troubles.

When Kim does a guest appearance for my Eat Clean™, Clean Living™ and Tosca Reno™ audiences, engagement is high, questions fly and women fall in love with her, just as I did. Women want to know how to stop the dribbling, pad wearing frustrations of weak pelvic floor health.

What Kim teaches in **Your Pelvic Floor** can be considered the ultimate user's manual to your vagina. You'd be surprised, for example, how visualizing a blueberry – as I learned to do – can help tweak your pelvic floor power. Don't worry! You'll find out.

Your Pelvic Floor demystifies pelvic floor health in a supportive and practical way that gives women of every age hope for a healthy relationship with their womanhood.

Tosca Reno
Tosca Reno is the *New York Times* best-selling author of *Your Best Body Now* and the *Eat-Clean Diet* series. She is a certified Nutritional Therapy Practitioner and a leading health and wellness advocate.

INTRODUCTION

How many times have you been to the dentist in your life? Chances are it is at least once, probably twice, a year from the time you were a child. You have been taught the importance of oral health, you brush your teeth twice a day, floss regularly and you have a check-up with your dentist even if you don't have any "issues", correct?

The same should be happening with your pelvic health. So, how many times have you been to a pelvic health physiotherapist…? Chances are, you've picked up this book because you are either under the guidance of a pelvic health physio, or you're reading up because you're experiencing pelvic floor dysfunction – whether that's incontinence, pelvic pain or prolapse – and you're trying to find healing tools. You've come to the right place. This book will be your guide through the problems we can face as owners of a vagina, and signpost areas to help you find the treatment programme that will be right for you.

The pelvic floor is a part of the body that deserves preventive health care, and education starting at around the time of menstruation. Function and pelvic health management strategies should be taught, along with education on the menstrual cycle. It is also important to inform vulva and vagina owners about *proactive* health care, and teach about things that can interfere with optimal function. Just like dentists teach that sugary foods and lack of brushing and flossing can lead to tooth decay and cavities, female health educators can introduce the concept that daily habits such as posture and the way you go to the toilet (yes, you read that right!), and life events such as childbirth can lead to challenges with your pelvic floor muscles.

Preventive health care just makes sense. Unfortunately, the healthcare system is more typically *reactive* and so many people are left feeling angry and resentful for not having been given the full picture earlier on. The 2020 results of the inquiry into the mesh scandal in the UK – where thousands of women were found to have been left in pain needlessly due to complications with unnecessary vaginal mesh surgery – display how women's health really needs to be higher up on the agenda, and for women's pain to be recognized and acknowledged – and alleviated – with more clarity and intention. Women risk feeling robbed of their opportunity to have made different choices, and may feel isolated, alone and frustrated when faced with a pelvic floor challenge that could have been prevented, managed or minimized with a proactive approach.

Then we feel lost in terms of what to do and are unaware of all of the options available to us. There exists an enormous amount of shame, confusion and embarrassment around pelvic health and there is thankfully a movement happening to make access to appropriate education and treatment standard care in the healthcare system, but it will take time for it to be fully adopted. We need to take matters into our own hands.

When your pelvic floor isn't functioning as it should, it may not be life threatening, but it is certainly life altering. You may start to plan outings based on available toilets. You might need to take extra time to get to work or maybe take more frequent breaks while at work. You may live in fear of other people knowing about the problem and go to great lengths to hide it: adopt the "incontinence uniform" of black leggings, multiple clothing layers and spare clothes in your bag at all times. You might begin to avoid social interaction or fitness altogether, for fear of having an accident. This begins to have an effect on relationships and intimacy, and can be incredibly distressing.

Shame, embarrassment and secrecy thrive in this atmosphere, you might not even tell your partner what's going on, which can create disconnection and a breakdown in communication. Many just ignore the leaks, laugh it off, wear pads and carry on. Indeed, we are conditioned to do this, with certain incontinence pad advert campaigns saying, "A little bit of wee won't stop me being me", advocating putting on a pad and just getting on with it, without exploring sorting the problem out.

Apart from the environmental impact of pads, this long-term dismissal of pelvic floor dysfunction does women no favours in terms of the impact of incontinence later in life. If we are fully informed then it becomes a matter of *choice* – the reality is so many people have no idea that *there is help*. Women suffer in silence, thinking we are the only ones, or that there is no solution. Some may recognize it as a problem, but are afraid or embarrassed to seek help. We might live in fear of making it worse and will reduce or avoid exercise which can in turn create a host of other health challenges, not to mention potentially worsening mental health aspects of dealing with the condition.

This book aims to offer coherent yet accessible information on pelvic anatomy and function, and its influence on whole body mechanics and well-being. This is a straight talking, taboo-shirking pelvic floor health guide. This is for *you* – the owner of *your pelvic floor* – who deserves to be informed and given resources that enable you to make informed choices about your physical, emotional and mental health. Information that is easy to understand and applicable to everyday life, along with easy-to-implement exercises that will help strengthen your pelvic floor, for life.

One in four women experience pelvic floor dysfunction and 2018 stats from NICE (the National Institute for Health and Care Excellence) suggest that 84% of pelvic floor dysfunction symptoms can be alleviated by pelvic health physiotherapy –

but up to 50% of people don't understand how to contract the pelvic floor correctly. Does this ring true for you?

Perhaps you've just had a baby and are noticing how important your pelvic floor is for the first time, now that it feels compromised. Or maybe you've been silently dealing with unwanted leaking, change in sensation or pelvic pain for years, and have finally had enough. Wherever you are in your pelvic health journey, this book is for you.

Pelvic floor muscle training improves muscle tone and so helps to prevent pressure on the pelvic floor in your daily movement (such as when you run, laugh, cough, pick up heavy objects), which helps to prevent incontinence. Verbal instruction to "go home and do your pelvic floor exercises" is not effective for everyone. There are also various forms of pelvic floor muscle training that extend beyond "kegels" but typically the only recommendation women get is to "do your pelvic floors" with no further guidance. Which can leave us feeling confused, embarrassed and deflated.

Pelvic floor dysfunction affects your physical health, your emotional health, your spiritual health, your relationships, your mood, your confidence. *You deserve to be informed.*

Your Pelvic Floor presents practical and physio-approved health, fitness and wellbeing tips along with advice from a variety of experts such as pelvic health physiotherapists, Pilates instructors, soft tissue therapists and doctors about the myriad benefits of strengthening your core and pelvic floor.

Pelvic health is not an easy topic for everyone to talk about. It can be associated with pain, trauma and shame, which then make it even harder to cope with. People are sadly often dismissed by their doctor when they seek help, and when you add on other considerations like a transgender experience, race, culture, religion and identity, this can make opening up these conversations even more difficult.

Pelvic health deeply affects our mental/emotional health, and if you're dismissed or not listened to, or feel ashamed of your symptoms, you may begin to withdraw from parts of your life. This might mean more sick days from work, not wanting to participate in group fitness classes, possibly avoiding social outings and withdrawing from partners or loved ones. Self-isolation and feelings of isolation are very common with pelvic floor dysfunction. This book can be your lifeline to make positive choices to change your pelvic floor health, and get your life back. Social media has played a significant role in increasing awareness and there are many private support groups online that are helping people seek help and guidance from others who are going through similar struggles. As awareness increases, people are finding the courage to ask questions, they are seeking out health care providers who listen and are beginning to work more collaboratively to ensure people have information and options.

It's important to mention that men have pelvic floors too, and do experience pelvic floor dysfunction. A lot of the information within this book is applicable to men: but this is explicitly a book written for the female/transgender, post vaginoplasty pelvic floor.

MY PELVIC HEALTH STORY

My pelvic health journey started in sixth grade when I saw a video about childbirth. It fascinated me but it also scared the heck out of me!

That video prompted me to ask my mom LOTS of questions, and thankfully she shared her answers very openly. As a medical professional (Operating Room Nurse) she was well informed and always made sure my brother and I were educated about our bodies by reading books with us, talking with us and answering our questions. I asked her about her birth stories. She told me that she had an episiotomy with both of her births and that pretty much confirmed for me that I was *not interested in having babies.*

Fast forward to when I was in university. My mum had a hysterectomy because she had fibroids and was bleeding heavily every month. Looking back, I now have so many questions and recommendations that may have helped her but at the time I simply accepted, as she did, that it was just what needed to be done.

A few years later she had surgery for incontinence. Again, I look back at that with the knowledge I have now and wonder if she could have avoided surgery had she known about pelvic health physiotherapy and the influence of her daily posture and movement patterns, or about hypopressives?

By this time, I had met my now husband and was starting to think that maybe I would like to start a family. In 2002 my sister-in-law gave birth and she allowed my husband and me to be in the room with her. Witnessing a woman giving birth assisted by midwives changed my whole perception of birth and the body. I was pregnant the following year.

My sister-in-law had done perineal massage and birthed in a side-lying position – something I had never seen before. I asked my midwives about their thoughts on perineal massage and if there was anything else I could do to prepare. One of my midwives told me about a biofeedback device called the EPI-NO that she felt may be helpful. I researched it, bought one and used it to prepare for both births. That decision was the spark that ignited my journey as the Vagina Coach and is ultimately what led me to now be writing this book.

I had a great birth experience, with no interventions or tearing. When sharing my story with others I was one of the few that had a positive birth experience. I realized then that there was no information widely available to pregnant people with regards to pelvic health. I decided to contact the manufacturer of the EPI-NO and ask if I could become a distributor.

I began preaching about the benefits of pelvic health physio not long after I started my business. Initially I was promoting it as something to help people who were dealing with incontinence and prolapse, but after seeing a pelvic floor physiotherapist myself (I had to practise what I was preaching) I learned that I had a prolapse. I began to recommend pelvic health physio in pregnancy, and for a comprehensive screening postnatally. Pelvic health physios can help assess for problems and ensure the inner workings of the pelvis continue to function optimally at all life stages.

It is now 2020 and I am writing this book in the middle of a pandemic. I feel incredibly grateful for my mother who was open to sharing her story, to my sister-in-law for allowing me to be present at her birth, for the EPI-NO and for being able to help so many people feel more confidence and heal their core challenges.

I am a cisgender woman whose work has primarily been with other cisgender women. I recognize that not all people with a vulva and a vagina identify as a woman, and I have done my best to use inclusive language throughout this book. However, much of the research I share, the client experiences and my personal story are with people who identify as a woman.

This book is a collection of my professional experiences with clients, published research and my personal stories, which I hope will inspire and empower you to put your pelvic health at the very top of your to do list. I am evidence informed and guided by physiotherapy best practice, but in this book I also share what I have personally seen work with my clients and myself, even when there is less clinical research to support it.

Every woman needs a vagina coach. I applaud you for choosing to educate and empower yourself with knowledge you can put into action right away. This book has been fully reviewed by a pelvic health physiotherapist and can offer you the essential groundwork for understanding, strengthening and appreciating Your Pelvic Floor.

Now it's up to you!

Kim Vopni

CHAPTER I
YOUR PELVIC FLOOR – A BIT OF ANATOMY

Understanding your anatomy is the first step in being empowered to strengthen your pelvic floor for the challenges of life. We are supported by our pelvis every day, but we probably give barely a thought to the muscles that provide our scaffolding in rest and movement. Here is a run-down of the key players in your pelvic floor health team. The pelvic floor doesn't work in isolation, like any good team, each player has a crucial role to play. There is more anatomy in the Appendix (page 151), if you'd like to read a bit more about the supporting muscular network.

The pelvis

Do you know where your pelvis is? You're most likely sitting on it now. It is the fulcrum of your balance, the shock absorber of all your movement. It's the turnstile through which your babies may have arrived, if you've ever given birth. Your pelvis is made up of two ilia (the bony parts you can feel at the front), two ischia (which form your sit bones, the bony parts of your bottom), all connected at the front to the pubic bone. The sacrum connects to the pelvis at the back, at the sacroiliac joints. The pelvis forms the scaffolding to which the pelvic floor muscles attach.

The pelvic floor

Your pelvic floor creates a springy muscular hammock spanning the pelvic cavity: providing support for your internal organs, and ensuring that your bodily fluids don't release (until you want them to).

The pelvic floor isn't one muscle but a collection of muscles, nerves, tendons, blood vessels, ligaments and connective tissue that are all interwoven into the bony pelvis. The pelvic floor is actually not one muscle but three layers of muscles that attach to the pubic joint at the front, the coccyx (tailbone at the base of the sacrum) at the back and the two sit bones on the sides. The pelvic floor provides the ability to close (to prevent your fluids and waste escaping) and lift (to support your organs in movement).

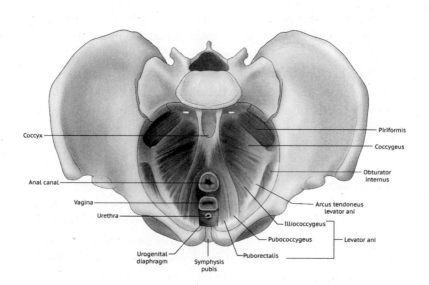

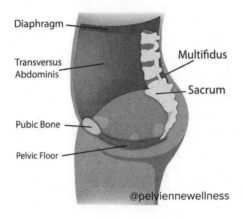

The core four

The pelvic floor is the foundation of the Core Four, the group of deep muscles responsible for stabilization and control of movement in your core. This group is made up of the pelvic floor, diaphragm, the transversus abdominis and the multifidus. Pelvic floor function is closely linked to your effective breathing, in creating tension in your abdominal wall and stabilizing your spine and pelvis.

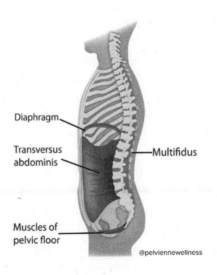

There are both "slow twitch" (approx. 65%) and "fast twitch" (approx. 35%) muscle fibres in the pelvic floor. Fast-twitch fibres are like the Olympic sprinters who act fast and tire quickly – these are the ones that prevent leaks when jumping, coughing, sneezing. Slow-twitch fibres are the endurance athletes, the marathoners who are slow and steady and don't tire as easily: this is your constant muscular support throughout the day.

The diaphragm and pelvic floor work together with the deep abdominals to help manage stability of the pelvis and spine – i.e. when you pick up your toddler or lift weights at the gym, your pelvic floor and lower abdominal network kicks in to support your spine and prevent leaking urine. We need the pelvic floor muscles to contract quickly, for example when we jump or cough, and we also need them for posture and control throughout the day.

The pelvic floor has many important jobs, which can be highlighted as the four Ss:

Stability – the pelvic floor plays a role in stabilizing and helping control the spine and pelvis.
Support – the pelvic floor plays a role in supporting the internal organs – the bladder, uterus and bowel.
Sphincteric – imagine like a gate that shuts: sphincters close tightly to stop anything passing. The pelvic floor is the gatekeeper in our continence.
Sexual – the pelvic floor is an essential part of your sexual response and pleasure.

The diaphragm
The diaphragm is your breathing muscle: the "roof" of your core, where the pelvic floor is the "floor". When you take a breath in, the diaphragm lowers down, the lungs expand which pulls air in. As you breathe out, the diaphragm rises back up as the lungs empty, moving air out of the body.

In an ideal functioning core, the pelvic floor moves synergistically with the diaphragm *with every single breath*.

- **When you breathe in**, the diaphragm lengthens and moves DOWN, and the pelvic floor also expands and lowers.
- **When you breathe out**, the pelvic floor contracts and lifts UP – as the diaphragm contracts and lengthens back up as well.

It is a beautiful synergistic dance between the two that happens all day long. In a nutshell: if you're mostly not breathing fully to allow your diaphragm to move, your pelvic floor also won't be functioning optimally. We will explore posture and alignment later on in the book (page 75).

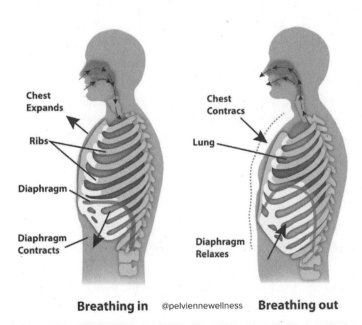

Breathing in   @pelviennewellness   **Breathing out**

The transversus abdominis

The transversus abdominis (TvA) is the deepest layer of the abdominal wall. It acts as a corset, stabilizing your spine and pelvis. It works together with the pelvic floor, and it helps with expelling air during a cough or a sneeze. Try it now: place one hand on your lower belly and make a little cough – you'll feel your tummy pull in momentarily.

The TvA moves inward and outward (toward and away from the spine). As it does, it creates the tension essential for "core control", to make your body withstand the loads placed on it day to day. This muscle must have varying amounts of tone throughout the day to help support the spine and the internal organs during movement and at rest. *Too much tone* can create a downward pressure on your pelvic organs, which may be a factor in incontinence and/or prolapse. Too *little* tone may lead to the inability to manage intra-abdominal pressure (for example, not stabilizing enough when forces are placed on your body, such as picking up a heavy object or getting up from the floor), which means there's a lack of support for the spine and/or abdomen.

The multifidus

The multifidus muscle runs down both sides of your spine, supporting the spine and pelvis, and also works in synergy with the pelvic floor and the TvA. Weakness in the multifidus can be a cause of back pain. Pain in the back or in the pelvis can start to create a pain–weakness cycle. The multifidus can become weaker or lose some of its elasticity due to postural habits, and that can lead to sacroiliac (SI) joint pain.

Whole-body movement and the pelvic floor

Optimal function of the pelvic floor means you are continent, pain free and moving well. Essentially, *if the pelvic floor is working well, you don't really think about it at all.* When the core is functioning optimally, your movement is anticipated, coordinated and balanced. When you bend over to pick something up, your body, your "core", knows you are doing that before you actually do it. It anticipates and prepares your body for that movement. It's this anticipatory action of your core that is so key to its optimal function. When things are going awry, it's often the anticipation that has been lost.

Remember: Our bodies are incredibly wise and give us messages we need to listen to. With a deeper knowledge of our inner workings, we can better understand *why* something may not be working as well as it could, and then find out *what* we may need to change in our daily life to heal.

HOW TO DO YOUR PELVIC FLOOR EXERCISES

If you're completely new to this, choose a position that will help you relax. Lying down, with your feet flat on the floor and knees bent, places less gravity force on the pelvic floor, so you *may* find it's easier to relax and find the right muscles. Ultimately, once you have found them, you need to practise in an upright position, sitting or standing, and then in movement, which will help strengthen your pelvic floor in a more "functional" way, that is – to make sure you are resilient for the movement of everyday life.

1   Take a deep breath in, relax your tummy and jaw.
2   As you breathe out, lift your back passage as if trying to hold in a fart. Travel that engagement forward, imagine stopping the flow of pee.
3   Hold that engagement, draw it up as much as you can without tensing your shoulders or buttocks.
4   Hold that engagement for a count of 5 – or as many seconds as you can hold the full engagement, building up to 10 seconds.
5   Let the engagement go and count to 5 as you breathe in and relax fully.

6 Repeat this 10 times: lift and hold for 10 seconds, release and rest for 5 seconds.

7 Try to remember to do this three times a day – but even once a day is a great start!

When you have found the muscles, you also need to practise faster lifts, which can feel trickier to master:

1 In a faster rhythmic pattern, holding for only one or two seconds: lift, squeeze, let go, squeeze, let go – ten times if you can.

2 Make sure you *release* fully in between the short, quick contractions.

3 Remember to practise both slow and faster contractions each day.

Ten long holds, ten short quick contractions, three times a day.

Now that you know how to find your pelvic floor – why not practise for a minute before you read the next chapter?

CHAPTER 2

THE SYMPTOMS OF PELVIC FLOOR DYSFUNCTION

So, what can go wrong with the pelvic floor? Understanding what "dysfunction" is will help you to realize when is the time to seek help and stop putting up with symptoms when you really don't have to. Your pelvic floor won't magically get better on its own, certainly not if you ignore what it's trying to tell you. It needs loving attention, support and guidance throughout life. Just like we all do! As you go through this chapter you may realize that you have been accepting symptoms as "normal" when actually they are worthy of investigation.

Incontinence

When urine leaks out of your body at any time other than when you want it to, it is considered incontinence. You may hear it called "light bladder leakage" or "sneeze-pee" or "peezing" but truth be told, pee coming out when you don't want it to is incontinence. It can be very distressing and life-altering, and it's a key factor in why elderly people are admitted to a care home. Knowing this, think about your future self: if you were to look back and realize *you didn't have to put up with incontinence* and you could actually make it better, what would you want to have done? What decision would you make for your body?

A lot of people will say, "Well, I only leak if I jump on a trampoline" or "I only leak if I run" and think that it is normal and do not consider themselves "incontinent". The reality is that *any unwanted urine loss at any time* is incontinence. While it is very common, it is not something you should accept as normal or something you need to live with. The good news is that it is very treatable.

Your bladder holds about 400–700ml of fluid (urine). At around 150–200ml you may get your first urge (or "signal") to pee and then as it fills up more you will feel a very strong urge. Tracking your urine volume (the amount) and symptoms and liquid volume intake is helpful when working to reduce or eliminate incontinence.

Completing a bladder diary is a great way to track your fluid input and output, as well as symptoms. I recommend doing it for three days, so you get a good idea of habits and possible food triggers. Having a measuring jug next to the toilet (that never makes it to the kitchen!) can help you track how much you are peeing, which you can then record in your bladder diary. A stop and start stream or difficulty starting the flow (if you are in a rush, or feeling as though you have to "push" to get it all out) can be signs of non-relaxing pelvic floor muscles, and possibly a bladder prolapse (which we will discuss in detail later on).

Keeping track of how frequently you urinate and what food and drink you have consumed during the day, can help you begin to notice potential bladder irritants or behaviours that could be contributing to your symptoms. Frequency is very much defined by the individual, but it's considered "normal" to empty your bladder once every 2.5–4 hours during the day. If you find that you are going more often you can use your bladder diary to determine if a food or drink may be irritating your bladder, if you are drinking a large amount of liquid in a short time or if you have some habits such as going to pee "just in case" before an exercise class or, for example, multiple times before leaving the house. With the awareness gained from using a bladder diary for three days, you can then make choices in food and behaviour that may help resolve the issues.

Stress urinary incontinence

If you experience urine loss when you laugh, cough, sneeze, run, jump, stand up from a chair … basically urine loss with any sort of exertion, it would be considered stress urinary incontinence. It can be a result of a breakdown in managing intra-abdominal pressure (for an explanation of this see page 26) that happens because of poor timing, meaning the pelvic floor is not able to "shut the gate" quick enough, or it can be a weakness issue, meaning the pelvic floor is not strong enough to "shut the gate completely", to prevent urine from leaking out.

Incontinence can also influence your balance. In one 2017 study,[1] 18 women with incontinence and 12 women without incontinence aged 50–55 years participated in two 60-second balance trials in four different testing conditions: eyes open/full bladder; eyes open/empty bladder; eyes closed/full bladder; eyes closed/empty bladder. The study found that the women with incontinence had more difficulty controlling their postural balance than continent women, while standing with a full bladder. This may support the desire or need of people to pee before every exercise class, but most people are doing this to avoid leaks rather than improve their balance. It is something you can test and observe in your own body. Exercises that require dynamic postural control may be easier with an empty bladder, but it's not ideal to use that as an excuse to go to the toilet if you don't really need to.

I feel it's important to point out that while the prevalence of incontinence increases with age – due to issues associated with menopause and decreased oestrogen, reduced mobility and dexterity, a more sedentary life – it is not *just* an ageing problem. Urinary incontinence affects 28% of women aged 30–39 and 55% of women aged 80–90. Other factors also can be at play with younger women, such as being overweight, depression, diabetes, pregnancy and birth, and hysterectomy are all associated with urinary incontinence.[2] Incontinence affects athletes as well. For elite athletes who've *not had children*, 28% have urinary incontinence; for trampolinists, it is 85%; gymnasts, 67%; and tennis players, 50%.[3]

One thing to note on statistics is that the numbers are based on *reported cases*. They don't take into account the huge number of people who suffer in silence and *never* seek help. Women wait an average of 7 years before seeking help, *if they do at all*.

Reasons for not seeking help include: not knowing the problem can be treated, thinking the only option is surgery, accepting the problem as "normal", feeling embarrassed or ashamed, and feeling uncomfortable approaching their healthcare provider.

Can you imagine the positive long-term effects if this information was shared with adolescent girls and young women when they first learn about sexual wellness? It could have a profound influence on the choices people make when seeking help, and I believe we would have more confidence about asking for help, including a better understanding of who to consult.

What is "intra-abdominal pressure"?

Intra-abdominal pressure (IAP) is the consistent pressure in the space between the diaphragm and pelvic floor. Intra-abdominal pressure fluctuates based on muscular resistance and whether you're breathing in, or breathing out. Where stress urinary incontinence is concerned, sudden increases in IAP create extra force in the abdominal area that your Core Four team can't manage, which results in leaking.

Our body is managing loads every day: external forces placed on it by movement, lifting, working against gravity, etc. The challenges occur when this pressure is not balanced and managed well. Some people adopt the strategy of avoiding activities that contribute to the greatest increases in pressure, which seems logical – but isn't realistic for daily life. Standing up from a chair (something we all do multiple times a day) actually creates more intra-abdominal pressure than a crunch exercise (curling your head and shoulders off the floor, using your abdominals), according to one study.[4]

A 2007 study[5] showed that holding your breath for a crunch increases IAP *more* than exhaling with the exertion, and that crunches have less IAP than a yoga downward dog. Coughing has nearly the same as jumping.

HOW DO I WORK *WITH* INTRA-ABDOMINAL PRESSURE IN MY DAY-TO-DAY LIFE?

When you cough or sneeze, or when you grab your fleeing toddler to put them in the buggy, these are the moments we are often caught off guard by our pelvic floor's failings. For these moments, we need to learn "the Knack".

WHAT IS "THE KNACK"?

In healthy pelvic floor muscles, not only do we need strong muscles, but they need to contract *at the right time*. This is one of our body's "reflexive" reactions, one that ideally we don't have to consciously think about – which is partly why we don't consider our pelvic floor to be important and vauable until something goes wrong. Where there is pelvic floor dysfunction, this reflexive contraction may have been lost. So we need to train it back. One way is with **the Knack.**

It has been shown that a well-timed, deliberate contraction of your pelvic floor can prevent leakage. Test yourself first. Do a strong cough, and see if you can feel your pelvic floor contract automatically *just* before you cough. If not, you need to practise "The Knack", which helps us to practise timing and coordination of our pelvic floor muscles.

This is how you do the Knack:

1   Make sure that you have been practising your quick, strong contractions that you hold for 2 seconds and release quickly. If not, go back to page 21 and find out how to do this.

2   Use this quick, strong pelvic floor contraction *just before* you cough, sneeze, bend, lift, or in any way are about to increase the pressure in your stomach (belly laughing will also cause this, hence the phrase, "I laughed so hard I peed my pants").

3   You need to consciously *and repetitively* practise the Knack until it becomes a "reflexive contraction" again.

4   One physio I know calls it "shutting the gate": consciously learn how to shut the gate before something escapes.

If you find over time that this reflex never gets retrained, so without consciously activating you still leak, take control and continue the Knack as a *regular habit*, to maintain good support and control of your pelvic floor muscles whenever you increase the pressure in your abdomen.

Practising the Knack regularly will help to retrain the reflexive reaction of your pelvic floor during activities that cause an increase in intra-abdominal pressure. So you need to practise this with: coughing, sneezing, lifting, bending over (particularly lifting *and* bending over, such as when you're lifting a small child), laughing and quick sudden movements.

We all have intra-abdominal pressure, we *have* to have it. There will always be things that create more or less of it, and even small levels of exertion will increase it to some degree. Therefore, suggestions to avoid certain activities or exercises because they contribute to an increase in IAP is perhaps not the best coping strategy. For example, you're told not to do crunches, but if you still get up out of bed every morning by crunching forward, it's better to learn how to manage that pressure properly.

The study also demonstrated that IAP is highly variable from person to person, even when performing the same task. Doing the same exercise, some people had very little increase in IAP, while others had greater increases. So it's important to consider an individualized approach to fitness, and ensure you have the right information to make informed choices about exercise and *your body*. Working with a pelvic floor physiotherapist is recommended. You may also benefit from seeking guidance from a Pilates teacher or personal trainer who has completed additional training in the pelvic floor.

Overactive Bladder

Do you constantly feel that you might need to go to the toilet, even if you've only just been? Are you always planning your day out around when you might need a loo visit and checking there will be facilities available?

You might find the urge to pee is triggered by the sight of your house, or being nearly home. Overactive bladder isn't always associated with incontinence, it can be wet or dry: so needs to be explored by a healthcare professional. You may begin to be anxious about travelling anywhere, which can really affect your quality of life and wellbeing.

Please visit your doctor if any of these resonate with you, as overactive bladder requires a regime of treatment from a professional rather than a "DIY" approach.

If you have a sudden urge to go to the toilet, which might appear "out of the blue" then you're suddenly desperate, this can turn into urge incontinence, which can be a symptom of overactive bladder.

Urge incontinence

Urge urinary incontinence is a bit less prevalent than stress urinary incontinence. It is characterized by a sudden urge to pee and can lead to a full release of the bladder. Many people will feel urges that correlate with certain activities, such as putting the key in the front door after arriving home, or as they get closer to the toilet after feeling a slight signal to go. Urge incontinence can sometimes be retrained working closely with a pelvic physiotherapist. Key techniques are managing fluid intakes and using a bladder diary. Timed voiding may also be successful, coupled with distraction measures. There is usually a period of 6 weeks of bladder retraining initially, and then medication may also be used. In conjunction with the bladder diary, you can become more aware of the frequency and your triggers. You can then choose to respond to the urges, or not. This can take time, and it's easy to become disheartened at the thought that it may take a long period of working with a pelvic health physio: but with commitment and dedication, urge incontinence can be managed and the frequency lessened.

If it has only been an hour since you last went and you are now feeling an urge, look at your diary: how much liquid did you consume in the last hour? How much before that? What type? Was there caffeine or was it something that could be considered a bladder irritant? If you have not consumed a large volume of liquid and haven't consumed anything that could potentially trigger the bladder then it's time to talk to your bladder. Walk to the toilet while talking to your bladder, but ideally, *you will not sit on the toilet.* Let your bladder know that you are aware of the signals, but that it is too soon to empty. Stand in front of the toilet and do some calf raises or curl your toes. You can also do some kegels. These are distraction measures that can help dampen the signal. Best practice is once you have calmed the urge, *then* you go back to the toilet, and pee. This is the first step in you taking back control.

Bladder training or timed release is best practised at home for a day or two and then you can use the strategies while at work or while out enjoying the day. *You don't have to talk out loud to your bladder*, obviously, this is something that may feel a bit woo woo and silly at first, but I do really recommend trying it as a strategy.

In an attempt to prevent leaking and/or urges to pee, many people start to go to the toilet "just in case", thinking that if there is nothing in the bladder then they won't get an urge or they won't leak: but here's the thing .... the bladder is *always filling*, and there is always a small residual of urine left. Emptying more often than needed will not solve the problem and can actually create other ones. "Just in case" peeing can mess with the brain/bladder messaging and does nothing to prevent leaks. It also trains the bladder to signal when it is not full, which can leave people feeling like they need to go all the time and the urges can become quite strong. We also have to be quite careful how we condition our children with this habit: "Make sure you go for a pee before we go out, just in case!" is not setting them up with good habits.

OAB presents a set of symptoms and urge incontinence is one of them. Detrusor overactivity can only be diagnosed by a test called urodynamics, so if you're worried, you will need to get tested and obtain a proper diagnosis and treatment plan. Medication is often necessary and is NICE recommended if six weeks of retraining does not work. It is important to work with a doctor and a pelvic floor physiotherapist to get a true understanding of what is causing the strong and frequent urges, so you can choose the right treatment solution to help to manage it.

Mixed incontinence

It is common to experience a blend of stress incontinence and urge incontinence. This would be considered mixed incontinence, and usually requires a blend of bladder retraining and pelvic floor muscle training in conjunction with a pelvic floor physiotherapist.

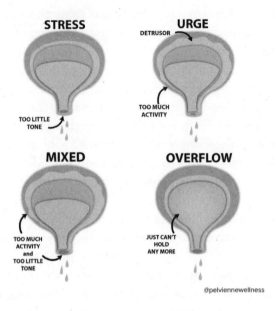

@pelviennewellness

Faecal urgency and incontinence

When people think of the word incontinence, they typically associate it with urine. However, uncontrolled wind and stool can escape the body at unwanted times with a loss of bowel control, which is called faecal incontinence.

While much less common than urinary incontinence, faecal incontinence can be devastatingly life-changing and impact hugely on sufferers' entire lives: work, relationships, self-esteem. One of the most common contributors to fecal, or anal incontinence, seen in women is obstetric anal sphincter injuries (also called OASIS). It involves damage to the anal sphincter, and in a fourth-degree tear (see page 80), the tear can get bigger and may even damage the lining of the anus or rectum.

If you are suffering from faecal incontinence, or faecal urgency (where you have the sensation of urgently needing a poo), you're not alone, you're not broken – *please* don't suffer in silence. There is support available, I have provided details of the MASIC Foundation (Mothers with Anal Sphincter Injuries in Childbirth) in the Resources section.

You can find help and put together a healing and management strategy working with a pelvic health physio. This can be really difficult to coordinate, often coinciding with life with a new baby, but it's truly worth it so please don't put it off any more. Pelvic floor exercises are a non-negotiable must for LIFE, consider it your essential daily maintenance along with brushing your teeth. I also recommend reading Luce Brett's book *PMSL – Or How Literally Pissed Myself Laughing and Survived the Last Taboo to Tell the Tale* for solidarity and support.

Vaginal wind

A close relative of unwanted wind from the anus is unwanted wind escaping from your vagina. Also known as – in the UK, anyway – "fanny farts". With "normal farts", you have an element of control and can clench your back passage and avoid it. With vaginal wind, it often takes us by surprise so you feel you aren't always able to prevent its escape – but a strong pre-emptive contraction of your pelvic floor usually works. It can happen during sex, or maybe when you're moving from an inversion such as downward dog in yoga – it can be horribly embarrassing. It may make an actual fart sound or just feel like bubbles escaping down there.

It's the result of trapped wind in the vagina, air being drawn into the vagina and then expelled, either as a result of penetration such as during penetrative sex or even a smear test, or upside-down movement such as some yoga poses, which draws air into the vagina. It can be caused by a variety of factors. If this is happening to you, please don't ignore it and put up with it, have it investigated as it can be a sign of something awry in your pelvic floor muscles, which can be treated with physiotherapy.

Pelvic organ prolapse (POP)

Around half of all women over 50 will experience a vaginal POP. You can have a prolapse without experiencing any symptoms, but a common symptom is incontinence. You may also experience pelvic pain, or a feeling of heaviness or "dragging", or as if something is stuck in your vagina, like a tampon which isn't in all the way. These symptoms definitely shouldn't be ignored.

The definition of pelvic organ prolapse is the descent and eventual protrusion of an internal pelvic organ into the vagina. The types of vaginal prolapse would be:

- **Bladder prolapse**, or cystocele, when the bladder bulges against the front wall of the vagina. It is also called an anterior wall prolapse.
- **Womb Prolapse**, or urethrocystocele, when both the urethra and the bladder bulge into the vagina.
- **Bowel Prolapse**, or rectocele, when the rectum bulges into the back wall of the vagina. It is also called a posterior wall prolapse.

I have a stage 2 rectocele and, at the time of writing this book, I have lived with it for over eight years. A rectal prolapse, which is different from a rectocele, is when the rectum protrudes through the anus. A uterine prolapse occurs when the uterus descends into the vagina.

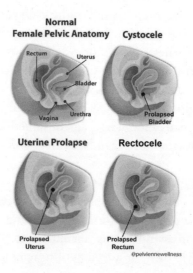

@pelviennewellness

Pelvic organ prolapse is typically graded 1–3 or 1–4, depending on what part of the world you are in. Typically, a grade-1 prolapse would be considered quite mild, where it's just starting to bulge ever so slightly into the vagina. Grade 2 would be considered moderate, where now it has descended and is getting close to the introitus, at the entrance to the vagina. Grades 3/4 are considered advanced and have a bulge at or out of the entrance to the vagina.

The presentation of a prolapse can vary throughout the day, so a prolapse could be a grade 1–2 in the morning and be a 2–3 by the end of the day. It varies with tiredness levels, bowel fullness, hormone cycle – it's important to be aware of the influence of the regular monthly flux of hormones, and understand that this affects prolapse and the presence of symptoms.

It can sometimes take 20 to 30 years for a pelvic organ prolapse to develop but it can also happen suddenly, such as during a heavy lift. Usually, it develops gradually over time and a lift or a sudden movement can be the straw that breaks the camel's back. Some other contributors to prolapse could be family history, chronic coughing and a high BMI. Posture has a huge influence as well: excessive rounding of the upper back has been shown to correlate with pelvic organ prolapse.

From a statistics perspective, 50% of women who have given birth have some degree of pelvic organ prolapse.[6] A more recent study showed that over 80% of women have some form of prolapse at 6 weeks postpartum, with over 50% of them having stage 2 or greater. It is incredibly common. Statistically it's more common than incontinence but so seldom talked about. A lot of women live with prolapse – and importantly, a lot of women live a full life and are able to manage their symptoms, to exercise and enjoy their life. So a prolapse doesn't need to be something that restricts your life.

Can prolapse be prevented?

This is a question that is hard to answer as there's no definitive evidence. Just as there is a huge missed opportunity for educating pregnant people about pelvic health in pregnancy, birth and postpartum recovery, there is a huge missed opportunity to educate people with incontinence and prolapse about prevention strategies and conservative treatment options and recovery practices *prior to surgery*. Arguably, if we knew how to look after our pelvic floor, and prioritized it – particularly around pregnancy and birth recovery, prolapse could be prevented.

Unfortunately, it is very common for people to have suffered in silence for years, and when they finally decide to seek help, they go to their doctor who refers them to a specialist, often a urogynaecologist, who then may start discussing surgery.

50% of women who have surgery for pelvic organ prolapse will experience a recurrence,[7] with 29% of those having a second surgery within two years.[8] Surgery generally eliminates symptoms associated with prolapse and can often restore anatomy – but it rarely addresses the causes of the problem. As a result, there is a very high likelihood of recurrence.

Surgery can be life changing and is *sometimes* the best choice – but without an understanding of the functions of the pelvic floor, posture, breathing, and movement strategies, people often find themselves needing to have surgery again because the root cause was never addressed. Many will say the surgery "didn't work" or "it failed". What failed is the holistic approach that was needed.

We need a village to manage our pelvic health and a collaborative approach between the medical community and pelvic health physiotherapists may serve people better in the short and long term by preparing the person for surgery (pre-hab), managing the post-op recovery (re-hab) and retraining core function to ensure the best possible and long-lasting surgical outcome.

Pelvic girdle pain (PGP)

Pelvic girdle pain (PGP) is typically associated with discomfort and/or pain in the joints of the pelvis. Pubic joint pain, typically referred to as symphysis pubis dysfunction, SI joint pain or coccyx (tailbone) pain are the most common. All are quite common in pregnancy but not unique to pregnancy. Often there will be a prescription of an SI belt that can sometimes be helpful in terms of relieving pelvic girdle pain and giving some support and stability to the joints in the pelvis as it becomes more flexible in pregnancy. It is important to note that wearing one when there is no indication of pain is not a beneficial practice as it can lead to muscles becoming dependent on the "help" of the belt.

From a statistics perspective, symphysis pubis dysfunction can persist postpartum in 7–10% of women. For some people, it won't bother them unless they are in aggravating positions such as standing on one leg, asymmetrical positions like lunges, getting out of the car or even rolling over in bed. About 45% of women will experience pelvic girdle pain in pregnancy, for 25% it will continue postpartum, and severe pain may affect about 8% of women.[9]

There are also pain syndromes that are not joint related and can be more challenging to diagnose and treat. Unfortunately, many people suffer for years before getting a true understanding of what they are dealing with because there is often nothing visibly wrong and no tests to help with diagnosis.

If you're experiencing pelvic girdle pain, please go to your doctor and arrange to see a pelvic health physiotherapist. Physiotherapy can do a lot to target the cause of pain.

Vulval/vaginal pain

Vaginismis and vulvodynia are two types of pain syndromes. Vaginismus is the experience of involuntary muscular spasms that can make penetrative sex difficult. Vulvodynia is persistent pain in and around the vulva and vaginal opening. Dyspareunia is pain during penetrative sex, and can be common in the postpartum period as it is sometimes related to perineal trauma and dryness. More on this on page 98.

Tearing during vaginal childbirth can be a contributor to pain. A second-degree tear (involving stitching) is likely to result in ongoing pain or painful sex, and third- and fourth-degree tears (requiring surgery) can be associated with an increase in pain, which should always be investigated.[10] Don't ignore vulval/vaginal pain – it is a sign that there is something wrong, it should be investigated so you can find a treatment and pain-management programme which can help. Try not to accept pain as a part of your life without questioning it.

What causes PGP and can it be treated?

Pelvic pain and pelvic girdle pain can have obvious causes like tearing or an episiotomy, but there can also be no apparent link to any injury or trauma. It may be a result of trauma to the perineum, but it could be a result of lack of strength or balance in the core muscles, which can cause an imbalance in the postural load on the pelvis. It could also result from hormone changes (dryness) and the ligament laxity that happens in pregnancy.

A common contributor to pelvic pain is overactive muscles, also called "hypertonic" pelvic floor muscles, which can result from poor posture, injury and non-optimal compensation strategies. From a treatment perspective, pelvic floor physiotherapy can be very beneficial and often focuses on soothing the nervous system and "down training": learning how to release overactive pelvic floor muscles which may be holding on to too much tension. SI belts may provide support to the pelvis and help decrease the pain. Once the pain is managed, sometimes the muscles can then work more effectively

Another pain syndrome that needs mentioning is bladder pain syndrome (BPS), also called interstitial cystitis (IC). It is a persistent condition of the bladder with no known causes. It can present with a variety of symptoms such as bladder pressure, bladder pain usually when the bladder is full, frequency (many are peeing small amounts frequently throughout the day and night), urgency and pelvic pain.

BPS can be difficult to diagnose, and often involves ruling out other treatable conditions before reaching a diagnosis of BPS or painful bladder syndrome. There is currently no cure for BPS, so the focus is on lifestyle management of the condition. For some oral or topical medications can help in combination with diet modification, bladder retraining, stress management and sleep. Pelvic health physiotherapy is also helpful in managing the symptoms associated with BPS.

CASE STUDY – KATHY (57)

Kathy came to me after being referred by a pelvic health physiotherapist who recommended me to help Kathy feel supported in her exercise regime and potentially try hypopressives (see page 117 for more on hypopressives).

Kathy had a very extensive history of pain – pelvic and lower extremity – and had seen multiple specialists including physios, pelvic floor therapists, massage therapists, Pilates instructors and doctors.

Her main goal when I met her was to get to the point of being able to hike pain free and potentially downhill ski again. She was also dealing with some urgency, and vaginal dryness.

Kathy gave birth to her first baby in 1987. It was a forceps-assisted birth. In 1990 she had her second baby and had second-degree tearing. In 1992 she had her third baby and again experienced tearing. In 2002 she had surgery for a rectocele repair as well as a sling for stress urinary incontinence. In 2004 she was active and doing body pump classes and began to experience piriformis pain, which became a very long road of various pain syndromes.

She emailed me a very extensive health history coupled with a Power Point presentation of her pain and treatment timeline. To be honest I was a bit intimidated but was up for the challenge. I approached her as I would any other client, and started with the basics.

When I met her for her first session she had all of her tools out and I knew she was dedicated and driven to feel better in her body. She had balls and bands and mats and release tools and had a daily practice. I first evaluated her standing posture and movement mechanics. She had developed some compensations and her posture was a key area to address. I gave her a few new release exercises including a standing hamstring release, a thoracic release and a calf release. I also taught her hypopressives and gave her one pose to practise until the next session.

I followed up with her a few days later and she said she already noticed a difference. She had done a spin class and all of the releases and hypopressives that I had given her and she had no pain – she was thrilled!

During her first follow-up session we chatted about her dryness and persistent UTIs. I suggested the possibility of food sensitivities so she made an appointment with a naturopath (NB – these types of options for management of your pelvic floor symptoms fall within "alternative" methods as opposed to evidence-based NICE-recommended treatments). She also began using a hyaluronic acid product for dryness and felt an immediate difference. I gave her a few more hypopressive poses to work on as well.

During her third session I fine-tuned some of the exercises she was doing and gave her three more hypopressive poses to do.

In the fourth session she was feeling much less pain and excited about her progress. She had gone hiking with no pain! She felt she was ready for more and she wanted to try one of my follow-along programmes. After a few days she was feeling worse, so when she reached out to me I recommended she stop and stick with what she was doing before. She had been feeling great initially and really wanting to increase the intensity, but soon found that she needed to progress much more slowly than she had anticipated. She was still very happy overall as she had made significant progress in reducing her pain and was enjoying more freedom in her life! She also welcomed a grandbaby and was preaching all about pelvic health to her daughter!

Lower back pain

Lower back pain (LBP) is typically pain in the mid to lower back. People describe it as a dull ache that's persistent, or possibly shooting or throbbing pain on occasion. It can lead to sciatica, and around 20% of people with lower back pain talk about the SI joint being the pain generator.[11]

In terms of contributors to back pain, it can often be brought back to the inner core having lost its ability to contribute to control, perhaps due to a loss of the anticipatory element or perhaps due to a muscle imbalance. When loads or forces are not transferred through the pelvis well it can result in altered movement and stabilization strategies that can then contribute to pain. In pregnancy, joint laxity may be a contributor as well as posture changes. The forward weight of the growing uterus and baby shifts the centre of gravity, which can lead to unconscious changes in posture to accommodate. The tailbone often tucks as the pelvis shifts forward and there is a loss of the curve in the lumbar spine, as well as an overactivation of the posterior pelvic floor muscles.

Swayback posture is also a common one in pregnancy, where the sacrum is held in a prolonged tilt that aggravates the SI joints. In pregnancy, the abdominal muscles may stretch beyond their optimal length and are often hindered in their ability to initiate and control movement, which can also contribute to pain in the lower back. Pain is an inhibitor of function, which can lead to weakness in the core, including the glutes and the pelvic floor.

One study showed that 78% of women with lower back pain have pelvic floor dysfunction, specifically urinary incontinence,[12] while another showed that 53% of women report lower back pain and pelvic girdle pain in combo.[13] More recently a group of Canadian researchers found that 95.3% of study participants were found to have some form of pelvic floor dysfunction. More specifically, 71% of the participants had pelvic floor muscle tenderness, 66% had pelvic floor weakness and 41% were found to have a pelvic organ prolapse. Participants with combined lower back pain and pelvic girdle pain presented with higher levels of disability and increased symptoms of pelvic floor dysfunction such as incontinence.[14]

Lower back pain is very common, especially with the increased amount of sitting we do as modern humans. Many seek help from an osteopath or massage therapist to manage back pain. Pelvic health physiotherapy may be the missing link for managing this bothersome condition. The benefit is that pelvic floor physio will address the cause of the back pain as well as the resulting pelvic floor challenges – win, win!

CHAPTER 3

WHAT CAUSES PELVIC FLOOR DYSFUNCTION?

When things are not working as well as they should it typically means symptoms start to show up such as pain, discomfort, tightness, constipation, incontinence, back pain and prolapse, which are the most common and referenced throughout this book. There are many contributors to pelvic floor dysfunction – and they are not always what you think.

When the pelvic floor is not working as it should, it can present in many different ways, and sometimes people can experience several types of core and pelvic floor dysfunction at the same time. Back pain, urge incontinence and bladder prolapse may all occur together, which can increase the mental health toll and may influence treatment, exercise solutions and lifestyle management. Just like there are many different presentations, there are also many different contributors to core and pelvic floor dysfunction. Knowledge about some of the more common ones can help highlight some that may be influencing you, as well as what you may be able to do to preventively or restoratively help reduce the likelihood of the development of or worsening of symptoms associated with incontinence, prolapse, back pain, etc.

The influence of posture

There is very little research on posture and its effect on pelvic floor muscle activity, symptoms and the development of dysfunction. Katy Bowman is a biomechanist and has been a leader in bringing to light body alignment for optimal core function.

She believes that as a society we are "outsourcing our movement" and that means our bodies are becoming de-conditioned and not accustomed to moving in a variety of ways, which then wreaks havoc on our overall alignment. The alignment of our head, shoulders, rib cage, pelvis and feet influences our ability to breathe, which directly influences our pelvic floor.

The postures we choose and live in for the majority of the time will create our alignment. Essentially, alignment is the by-product of our posture. Another way to look at it is that posture is how we look and alignment is how we work. Our muscles adapt to how we hold our skeleton and with the increased amount of sitting we do, it is becoming more common to see posterior pelvic tilt and a loss of the curve in the lower back – this will impact on the depth of our breathing, and, as we've seen, this affects our pelvic floor function.[1]

It's okay to slouch every now and then, but it's not the posture we should live in for the majority of the time. Otherwise, our resulting alignment will start to influence our function. It is common, especially in today's world where we are constantly on our phones, to see a lot of people with forward head, "text neck", and rounded shoulders. With this posture it is also common to experience gripping in the upper abdomen, which can increase IAP. This gripping is often a compensatory strategy the body finds to try and control the core, and can be a reason why many people (postnatal women in particular) experience a roundness in their tummy if it is usually "flat".

Another common posture is to a forward thrust of the pelvis, with a loss of the lumbar curve in the lower back. There is often a posterior tilt of the pelvis and gripping in the buttocks that can lead to pain and a non-relaxing "hypertonic" pelvic floor that is less able to respond to increases in IAP.

An overactive pelvic floor

A contributor to stress urinary incontinence is overactive pelvic floor muscles that are fatigued and are not able to generate a maximal contraction because they are in a partially contracted state for the majority of the day. It essentially means that when the pelvic floor is needed during a sneeze or cough or jump, it's not able to respond appropriately and strongly enough because it is fatigued. Observing and learning about your postural habits, and developing an awareness of the position of your ribs over your pelvis, pelvis over your ankles may help you in your quest to heal pelvic floor challenges such as incontinence and prolapse.

MIRROR, MIRROR

Only when you truly see yourself in your comfortable patterns, can you look to noticing what it might be that could be influencing your muscle balance.

- Have a look at yourself in the mirror now, in your natural standing position. Maybe even get a friend or partner to take a picture of you standing, from various angles: from the front, side, behind.
- Really observe the way that you hold your body, the familiar shape of your posture as you carry yourself day to day.

To adjust your posture into a more "ideal" pattern will feel unfamiliar and slightly weird at first. Stick with it, your pelvic floor will thank you!

Protective postures

Many people with prolapse have unknowingly developed overactive pelvic floor muscles because they are afraid their organs will fall out. Or perhaps you've had abdominal surgery, and have developed compensatory posture to protect your abdominal wound, which has become your "normal". You might have adopted a gripping strategy as a way to feel like they are preventing your prolapse from worsening, when in actual fact you may benefit more from learning to let go and release that tension and then train the pelvic floor through its full range of motion. Notice if you're "tucking your pelvis" constantly and flattening your lower back: one study found that a loss of the natural lumbar curve appears to be a significant risk factor for the development of pelvic organ prolapse.[2]

Footwear

Ankle position can also have an influence on pelvic floor muscle contraction. One study looked at pelvic floor muscle contractions in three different positions – dorsiflexion (with the toes drawn toward the shin), neutral and plantarflexion (the ankles pointed away from the shin). There was significantly greater pelvic muscle activity with the ankles in dorsiflexion.[3]

If we consider the footwear that many people wear, most have a positive heel, meaning the toes are lower than the heel (plantar flexion), which the study showed resulted in decreased pelvic floor muscle activity. Spending more time barefoot or in neutral heel shoes, especially during standing positions, while doing pelvic floor muscle training, could potentially play a role in reducing symptoms and improving pelvic floor function. Releasing tension in your feet by massaging over a tennis ball is a good way of counterbalancing the effects of your daily posture.

When you think about this in relation to a pregnant body, maybe the saying "barefoot and pregnant" is something we should pay more attention to. Pregnancy is often a contributor to the rounding shoulders, the gripping of the ribs and buttocks and the forward thrust of the pelvis. If a pregnant woman then wears positive heeled shoes, it will mean more plantar flexion and the resulting accommodations the body needs to make, on top of the ones it is already making to manage the ever-growing baby, will exacerbate the potential hip thrust and bum gripping that is messing with the alignment.

Considering your movement patterns in relation to your posture and your footwear can be a really valuable way of noticing what factors you have control over, when it comes to taking ownership of your pelvic floor health.

Ageing

We all age, and for those of us who have the privilege of living a long life there may also be more opportunities to be faced with a pelvic floor challenge. Each year that passes means more time against gravity, potentially more bone loss or muscle loss and more collagen loss. Perhaps it was a highly stressful year or one where you were sitting more often than in previous years.

A sedentary lifestyle is a risk factor for female urinary incontinence, so by avoiding movement for fear of making it worse, people are actually worsening their incontinence. There can be one single life event that suddenly changes your body's resilience. Maybe you were in a car accident or had a fall. Maybe you became pregnant or gave birth. Menopause is one life event which gradually impacts on pelvic floor health for many women. We are all faced with many different life experiences that also coincide with the fact that we age.

Ageing is inevitable, and pelvic floor health is known to decline with age; this is one of those fundamental truths. But, just because we age and each face many of the things mentioned above, does not mean we should give up or that things can't get better. Supporting our bodies and pelvic health as we age is hugely beneficial. Your pelvic floor will always respond to loving attention and care.

Doing pelvic floor exercise (such as kegels) incorrectly

Pelvic floor exercises are often prescribed but rarely taught so as a result, many people are doing them incorrectly. Some will squeeze their glutes, some will squeeze their inner thighs, some will sort of suck in and up on an inhale while others will hold their breath and bear down – something called a Valsalva manoevre. A Valsalva is essentially a somewhat forceful exhalation against a closed airway which can increase pressure. A proper pelvic floor contraction demonstrates more activity in the pelvic floor muscles when compared with a Valsalva.[4]

Pelvic floor rhythmic muscle contractions are also known as kegels. The kegel exercise was invented by Dr Arnold Kegel, an American gynaecologist who noticed that his female patients were experiencing difficulty with their pelvic floors after childbirth. He used the perineometer, which was a tool designed to measure the contraction and relaxation of the pelvic floor muscles. The feedback was shown on a gauge and helped the people see the action of their muscles, which was good education and also good motivation.

Dr Kegel undertook an 18-year medical study and eventually published a paper in 1948 called "A Nonsurgical Method of Increasing the Tone of Sphincters and Their Supporting Structures". He noted how much difficulty many of his patients had in doing kegels correctly and found the visual control offered by the perineometer was helpful. By 1950 his cure rate was impressive – over 90% – which is why this exercise is still very much in use today. The challenge has been that many health care professionals make assumptions on a person's ability and knowledge. People benefit from a thorough pelvic floor assessment and education on how to properly recruit and relax the pelvic floor muscles.

How do I learn how to "do my pelvic floors" correctly?

A pelvic health physiotherapist is considered the gold standard for assessing and treating the pelvic floor; however, not everyone has access to one. As an alternative, there are great biofeedback products on the market that can offer some assistance for those who are not able to see someone in person. Devices can also be helpful alongside seeing a pelvic health physiotherapist. The gamification aspect of some of the devices is motivating and engaging, and helps with consistency.

Using pelvic tech

The Elvie is a popular choice and the technology can also decipher between a person who is engaging the muscles correctly and someone who is bearing down. This is the one I recommend most. Another is the Perifit and finally, the EPI-NO, which is extra beneficial for use in pregnancy because it can help with perineal massage and learning to yield to sensations of stretch and pressure.

Once someone is doing pelvic floor exercises *correctly*, there are two additional elements that will make them effective:

1   They need to be done *consistently*
2   They need to be *coordinated* with movement.

This is my 3C approach to pelvic floor fitness and I will elaborate more on this in the fitness section (see page 127).

Hormones

The influence of hormones is constant and changes as we progress through different life stages. We will cover the main hormones in pregnancy in the next chapter (see page 69), and it is important to note that some people give birth and then may actually be perimenopausal. Perimenopause is the period of usually 6 to 10 years prior to menopause, and menopause is the day that marks one year without periods. That's right – "the menopause" is technically just one day. Leading up to it is considered perimenopause and after that one day is considered post-menopause. With more and more women choosing to become pregnant later in life, some women may be perimenopausal when they become pregnant.

Oestrogen fluctuations postpartum and during peri- and post-menopause are a contributor to vaginal dryness. It affects the tissue elasticity, lubrication and can contribute to decreased tone in the pelvic floor. Many women report that they've never had any leaking or pelvic floor challenges before, but as they get closer to menopause or even post-menopause, all of a sudden those issues become apparent. Progesterone influences the mood and the sense of wellbeing, and it's often the imbalance between oestrogen and progesterone that causes challenges.

Menstruation

Closely aligned with hormonal flux, your cycle affects your pelvic floor. So it's really important that you begin to track your cycle and chart how your symptoms show up, and where, within your cycle. We have been given this amazing rollercoaster of hormones, we might as well learn to ride it and harness their power.

One study showed that 41% of women notice that their incontinence is cyclical, and of those women, 42% experience symptoms just before their period and 36% of women notice increased symptoms during their period.[5] What this means is that approximately a week before menses occurs there is a drop in oestrogen, which is believed to decrease the strength of the urethra, the tube that connects that bladder to the urinary meatus (how we get urine from the bladder to the outside).

The pelvic organs, as well as the surrounding connective tissues, are all oestrogen-responsive, meaning the tissues respond and adapt to fluctuations in oestrogen. This is something to pay attention to as it gives us a glimpse into what we will face once we approach and reach menopause, when oestrogen levels decline significantly.

When it comes to the seasons of our cycle, here is where I tend to personally lean toward alternative and intuitive practices, which are currently without solid evidence-base in terms of robust clinical research for pelvic floor health. It's always worth exploring the treatment that works for *your* body. And investigate options that resonate with you personally, as well as consulting a professional pelvic health practitioner.

Many people notice an increase or worsening of symptoms just before and during their menstrual cycle. This is thought to be because of fluctuating hormone levels, in particular declining oestrogen. Being aware of the influences of hormones on the body, in particular the pelvic floor, can help you understand your moods, cravings and energy levels and also allow you to cycle your workout intensity based on the phase you are in. The average cycle is between 26 and 35 days, with 28 days being the most typical. Each phase within your cycle brings something different.

Days 1–7 Menstruation

Days 1–7, when you are bleeding, are also called the Early Follicular Phase. During this time the body sheds the lining of the uterus. Many report feelings of tiredness, back ache, cramps and generally wanting to retreat. Yin-focused activity is very nourishing to the body during this time. An example of "yin-focused activities" would be restorative yoga or yin yoga, meditation, long walks and passive release-type stretches and poses. It is a time to down-regulate, hibernate and in essence start planning for the next phase. Knowing that many are more symptomatic during this time with regards to their pelvic floor, it is helpful to acknowledge that the larger uterus may be at play and that hormones are at their lowest, which can affect the contractile tissue in the body.

Days 8–14 Follicular Phase

Days 8–14 are considered the Late Follicular Phase and it is a time when energy is rising. Oestrogen is also rising, which can actually help build muscle faster as it speeds repair and regeneration of muscle tissue. Short cardio sessions, and high rep/low weight resistance training would be good exercise options during this phase.

Days 15–20 Ovulation

Ovulation marks days 15–20 and is when you may feel your most energetic and powerful. Testosterone and oestrogen are at their peak so take advantage with higher intensity workouts, higher resistance, lower reps and higher impact and endurance exercise. Progesterone is also higher, which helps the body become more efficient at using fat for fuel. It may be tempting to really "go all out" with higher impact workouts when you're feeling energetic, but make sure you notice and track your pelvic floor symptoms alongside increased impact with your exercise.

Days 20–28 Luteal Phase

Oestrogen is now starting to fall and some will feel unmotivated and tired, perhaps even struggling with PMS. Progesterone and testosterone are also falling, which shifts you out of muscle-building mode. Focusing on muscular endurance workouts that are low impact is best and helps manage or offset any potential increase in symptoms. The uterus is increasing in size and weight as it prepares to shed its lining (or grow a baby). The average normal weight of the uterus is 2.5 ounces and that increases up to three times during menstruation. A bigger, heavier uterus could definitely contribute to an increase in symptoms, especially prolapse.

Endometriosis

An estimated one in 10 women suffer with this often-debilitating disease and unfortunately it can take on average eight to ten years before it is properly diagnosed. Before people with endometriosis are diagnosed, they are often told they have dysmenorrhea – painful periods and PMS "cramps" – and given painkillers to help manage their symptoms. But the condition is not as simple as "painful cramps".

Endometriosis is characterized by the presence of tissue from the lining of the womb, found outside of the uterus. This tissue forms lesions that contribute to pain and inflammation, with some of the more common symptoms being crippling period pain in people who menstruate, pelvic pain, painful intercourse, leg and lower back pain, fatigue and bowel/urinary dysfunction, to name a few.[6]

The condition often starts at an early age and most typically begins in the pelvic tissues. It can contribute to infertility and it is often not until a person is open to conceiving that it leads to a diagnosis of endometriosis. Of the teens who have pelvic pain, 70% go on to be diagnosed with the condition later in life.[7] There are many theories as to what causes endometriosis but no definitive answers. Many believe people are born with the condition and a combination of influences trigger the disease later in life.

There are no blood tests or biomarkers that diagnose the disease. The only way to definitively diagnose endometriosis is through a laparoscopy, which is also a treatment as well. Laparoscopic excision, also known as LAPEX, is considered the gold standard for treating endometriosis but not all surgeons are trained in this technique.

Pelvic health physiotherapy can benefit those suffering with endometriosis by helping improve the function of the muscles in the pelvic floor that are often affected by endometriosis. They do not treat the condition but rather help manage the symptoms associated with it. Abnormal muscle tension often develops in response to pain and becomes a secondary source of pain that can lead to painful intercourse and other forms of pelvic pain.

Treatment with a pelvic health physiotherapist may include manual therapy, modalities like ultrasound, ice or heat, education and stress management tips and potentially biofeedback. Heba Shaheed is a pelvic floor physical therapist in Australia who suffered with severe pelvic pain starting in her teens. Her search for solutions allows her to now help others. Some of her top recommendations include avoiding gluten and sugar, eating leafy greens and cruciferous vegetables, yoga, deep breathing and pelvic floor relaxation exercises. She specializes in complex female pain and endometriosis in her practice. See her top tip in the Pelvic Health Village section at the end of the book.

ADENOMYOSIS: MY STORY

I had never heard of adenomyosis until I decided to investigate why my periods were getting heavier and more painful, and why I was passing very large clots with each cycle. I had a pelvic ultrasound and it showed an "abnormally thick uterine lining" as well as an ovarian cyst. I then had a uterine biopsy to rule out cancer, and was told to wait a month to see if the cyst went away. It did and my biopsy came back negative. I was offered birth control to help manage my bleeding. I declined and continued on my journey.

I asked my doctor to check my hormones. Everything came back normal ... except my iron, which was alarmingly low; this was not surprising given the amount of blood I lost each month. I began reading books on hormones and then decided to pay for a more robust hormone test done through my naturopath. The results showed high estrogen and low progesterone along with adrenal fatigue. I started on bio-identical hormones and noticed some improvement but again, not significant. I had another pelvic ultrasound and again had the abnormally thick uterine lining. My doctor then suggested an MRI to confirm adenomyosis. Confirmed.

Adenomyosis is defined by the presence of endometrial tissue found within the muscular wall of the uterus, the myometrium, and typically leads to heavy bleeding, painful periods and often a distended abdomen.[8] My naturopath suggested an IUD (intrauterine device, or coil). I was reluctant given I was working to balance my hormones and didn't want something else to interfere. I also wasn't keen on something inside of me. "It isn't natural," I said. "It isn't natural to lose half your body weight in blood each month either," my naturopath responded. So I decided to try an IUD, the Mirena. Many people with an IUD cease having periods. That wasn't the case for me, although it did definitely help.

I kept reading about hormones and found my symptoms were closely associated with hypothyroidism. I then learned about an autoimmune condition called Hashimoto's that presents very similarly to hypothyroidism and results in many people being misdiagnosed and put on thyroid medication. I asked my naturopath to do a full thyroid panel blood test. Remember here that this is my personal experience, and one that led me to experience changes within my cycle and my own symptoms. It is not necessarily advocated by NICE guidelines in terms of treatment.

The important part of a complete thyroid panel is the antibodies. My results came back with elevated antibodies and while it was not enough to diagnose me with Hashimoto's, all things were pointing to me being on my way to an autoimmune condition.

My reading had told me that gluten was the first thing that needed to go. I had dabbled in gluten free but had never truly eliminated it. Once it was gone my symptoms definitely improved. I then began reading about the gut and about inflammation. I did food sensitivity testing to find out what else may be contributing to an inflammatory response in my body. Dairy, eggs and flax. I removed those and the improvement in my symptoms was remarkable! I had no more bloating or cramping, the length of my bleed lessened, the clots were gone and the few rectocele symptoms I had were gone. It was life changing. I still bled more than the average person and I would still experience flooding on occasion, but nothing like I used to. I would fill up a super plus tampon in 20–40 minutes for the first two days of my period and then bleed for an additional seven to ten days. Every month! Once I changed my diet my bleeding started to regulate. I was getting my life back!

I began writing this book during the Covid-19 pandemic. I would sometimes get a histamine reaction to red wine and so I stopped drinking wine… and my periods completely normalized. Completely! NO cramps, NO bloating, five to seven days of normal bleeding. No flooding. Life changing!

I share my experience in hopes that it may help you. Advocate for yourself, go to your doctor, read, seek alternative healthcare if that is the right option for you, stay open minded and be patient. This took years and it really shouldn't have. I am grateful for those who helped and that I was determined to figure it out and get to the root cause.

So, was it adenomyosis? Or was it that I had a lot of inflammation in my body and bleeding was my body's reaction? Heavy bleeding, painful cramps and clots are often disregarded as simply "normal" as you approach menopause, but I believe they are signals the body is sending asking for help. **The key is to do your research and seek care from those who will support your quest to address the root cause.**

Menopause

Menopause is one day. You officially reach menopause 12 months after your last period. Beyond that you are considered post-menopausal. Many people find that they have an increase or an onset of pelvic floor dysfunction symptoms when they reach the menopausal years. It can be difficult to determine if this is age related or menopause related. The main contributor to the development or exacerbation of symptoms associated with pelvic floor dysfunction is thought to be the decline of oestrogen. There are oestrogen receptors in the tissues of the vagina, in the pelvic floor muscles and in the uterosacral ligaments. Declining and low levels of oestrogen in perimenopause and post-menopause may affect the collagen in these tissues, which can result in dryness and atrophy. The term Genitourinary Syndrome of Menopause (previously known as "vaginal atrophy") is now used to describe the common symptoms of pelvic floor changes associated with this stage of a person's life.

As we approach menopause, the ovaries are starting to shut down and because they're a source of hormone production, we need to pull from other sources. The adrenals are typically where the body goes to for hormone-production assistance. When you think about how much stress and busy-ness and craziness we have in our lives, and how many people are dealing already with adrenal fatigue, relying on the adrenals for assistance with hormone production is not ideal.

It is also important to note that menopause is itself, a stressor. It is something that people dread and worry about, which contributes to an increase in cortisol production. When there are higher levels of cortisol, it encourages muscle breakdown so that there's more glucose to provide to the brain. This works against us with regards to our overall muscle tone and the form and function of our bodies. Elevated cortisol levels also increase blood sugar, which leads to cravings. People often eat a bit more, move a bit less, and the excess energy is stored as fat. There's often more visceral and belly fat that women gain as they approach menopause.

Post-menopause there is a decline in testosterone, which contributes to a lower sex drive and decreased muscle mass. With the weight gain and the appearance or worsening of pelvic floor symptoms, many women want to work out harder. This can create further elevations in cortisol and potentially a worsening of pelvic floor symptoms. Many people stop exercising as a result and with the reductions in bone mass that also accompany menopause, it puts people at greater risk of fractures and osteoporosis.

Hysterectomy

Hysterectomy is the second most frequently performed surgical procedure (after cesarean section) for women in the United States. Data from the UK suggest a rate of 42/100,000 population, while Canada is 108/100,000. Countries with no waiting times for surgeries have even higher rates, with Germany reporting rates of 236/100,000 and Australia 165/100,000.

According to the Centers for Disease Control and Prevention, from 2006–2010, 11.7% of women between the ages of 40 and 44 had a hysterectomy.[9] By the age of 60, more than one-third of all women have had a hysterectomy. Many doctors report hysterectomy as having been the standard procedure for many years, and many people believe that surgery is the only option, but thankfully a decline in this belief in the medical community is starting to happen as younger doctors become more aware of less invasive options to try first if the reason for hysterectomy is not life threatening. The most common, non-life-threatening reasons for a hysterectomy are prolapse, heavy periods and fibroids. Many women believe that surgery is their only option but thankfully, as physician awareness increases, knowledge about pelvic floor physiotherapy increases and as more women share their stories with one another, more people are investigating the root causes prior to jumping right to surgery.

Endometriosis, adenomyosis and fibroids are very common contributors to heavy bleeding, which is one of the reasons a woman may be advised to have a hysterectomy or choose to have one. Hysterectomies are not a cure for endometriosis. They may be considered a "cure" for adenomyosis but I believe many women with adenomyosis are given the option of a hysterectomy, which sounds amazing when someone is suffering, however it does not address the root cause of the condition and can leave people more at risk of other pelvic floor dysfunctions.

Another common contributor to heavy bleeding is hormone imbalance, specifically oestrogen dominance. Oestrogen dominance doesn't always mean "too much oestrogen", but rather a discrepancy in the ratio between oestrogen and progesterone. If someone is low in progesterone, they can in turn be oestrogen dominant. There are so many things that can lead to a disruption in the balance between these hormones such as inefficiency in removing excess estrogen, poor diet, exposure to endocrine disruptors, environmental toxins, stress, lack of sleep, hypothyroidism, Hashimoto's disease and even dehydration.

During perimenopause as the body prepares for menopause, estrogen levels decline and because there are fewer ovulations, there is also less progesterone produced. This also tends to be a stressful time of life and many people struggle with blood sugar balance and high cortisol levels. When we are stressed, our body makes more cortisol, and when the stress continues the body can't keep up with the demand so it starts to steal from other hormones. The stressed-out adrenal glands will use progesterone to make more cortisol, which contributes to the oestrogen/progesterone ratio being out of balance. This was me.

Thankfully I was curious and sought out multiple opinions and healthcare providers, something I know not everyone has access to – but more importantly most people don't even know there are other options. The medical community is typically the first line of defence when we feel that something is not right in our body. We absolutely need a great doctor as part of our healthcare team, but they don't always present more holistic options such as diet and lifestyle changes, or hormone and thyroid function tests. This results in many people possibly having an unnecessary hysterectomy.

There are a few different types of hysterectomy.

- A partial hysterectomy (also called a subtotal hysterectomy or a supracervical hysterectomy) involves the removal of the upper part of the uterus while leaving the cervix in place.
- A total hysterectomy removes the entire uterus and the cervix.
- A radical hysterectomy removes the entire uterus, the cervix and the top part of the vagina.

A decision will need to be made about the ovaries and fallopian tubes as well. Once the uterus is removed periods will cease. If the ovaries are also removed this will induce a surgical menopause, which means you will lose the protective effect of oestrogen as it relates to osteoporosis, heart disease and dementia.

There are a few different ways hysterectomies are performed, with vaginal surgeries being less invasive and more common. Vaginal hysterectomy and laprascopic hysterectomies often have faster recovery times, shorter hospital stays and even a reduction in pain and scar tissue.

Scar tissue is one aspect of the potential negative effects of a hysterectomy. Adhesions are a build up of scar tissue that can become sticky almost like Velcro, and can attach to your internal organs and interfere with the ability of the muscles to contract and relax. They can also cause tissue restrictions that may contribute to pain. Another consequence of hysterectomy is the removal of the "keystone organ", and disruption to the tendons and ligaments around the vagina and uterus. When the uterus is removed, it alters the surrounding support mechanisms which can contribute to the development of a vaginal vault prolapse (when the top of the vagina starts to collapse in on itself) and enterocele (when the intestines herniate downwards due to lack of support from the uterus).

As awareness about pelvic floor health increases and in hopes that there will be more collaboration between pelvic health physiotherapists and doctors, perhaps the rates of hysterectomy will decline. There are of course reasons why a hysterectomy has to be done, for example with cancer, and there will be people who choose to have a hysterectomy either after trying the non-invasive methods or not wanting to try them. Informed choice is the goal. Informed about options, informed about risks and informed about recovery and the increased risk of prolapse. This would hopefully give them the knowledge about what to look for in their own bodies and lifestyle choices as well.

Family history

Heredity is a risk factor for the development of prolapse. One study showed that the risk of prolapse was 1.4 times higher in women with a family history of prolapse and/or hernia.[10] Women are also more likely to experience incontinence if their mothers and older sisters experience incontinence.[11]

We can learn a lot from our mothers and aunts and grandmothers. Knowing their health history and watching what they experience can give you a leg up in terms of prevention. Knowing you are predisposed to pelvic floor challenges puts you in a position of power. You can make choices and put your awareness to work. Just because your mom or sister or aunt or grandmother had incontinence and/or prolapse doesn't mean you will. Especially if you take a proactive approach to your pelvic health.

Connective tissue disorders

Joint hypermobility is a common aspect of connective tissue disorders such as Marfan syndrome and Ehlers-Danlos syndrome (to name a few). Hypermobility essentially means an increased range of motion at the joints and is thought to be about 70% heritable, and seemingly more common in females.

These disorders contribute to changes in collagen that can significantly increase the risk of stress urinary incontinence and pelvic organ prolapse. People with these conditions may also be more sensitized to symptoms.

Obesity and a sedentary lifestyle

A Body Mass Index (BMI) of equal to, or greater than 25 is an established risk factor, at least for posterior prolapse.[12] It is widely agreed that obesity is linked to the development of urinary incontinence and organ prolapse and that weight loss can help reduce symptoms associated with these challenges.[13] [14]

The BMI can be misleading because people with more muscle mass can appear to be obese according to the BMI. For those who are overweight or obese, factors such as medications, diet, activity level and other diseases need to be considered as well. Some medications can contribute to constipation, some may contribute to weight gain, some may irritate the bladder. Diet may be a contributor to becoming overweight or obese and often sugary inflammatory foods are a culprit. Too much sugar can contribute to inflammation, and inflammation can often trigger symptoms.

Lack of exercise or a generally sedentary lifestyle may be a contributor to being overweight, and perhaps it was fear of making an existing pelvic floor challenge worse that led to the cessation or reduction of exercise. Lack of varied movement is a risk factor for so many things, and also leads to poor posture and a sedentary body that is not moving nutrients, blood and lymph as needed. A blend of nutritional advice and movement is an essential part of reducing body weight, which can in turn help improve symptoms associated with pelvic floor dysfunction.

High-impact exercise

In the last several years as the awareness about diastasis recti and pelvic floor dysfunction has increased, so too has opinions on movement and exercise. In the early years of my work there was very little research, and as pelvic health physiotherapists and fitness professionals began to collaborate there was a lot of "good" and "bad" exercise lists created. Soon the "bad" or "avoid" list became quite extensive, and so many people were barely moving for fear of making their condition worse.

The body needs to move.

We benefit from exercise in so many ways, and avoiding it or working in a limited range of movement may not be as protective as once thought and could perhaps contribute to other non-optimal compensations.

Running

Running is incredibly high impact on your pelvic floor. You have the force of gravity going down, and the ground force going up with each foot strike, meeting in the middle at your pelvic floor as the shock absorber. For those runners who depend on running for that "runner's high" (and I was one of them for years), the idea of stopping running is unthinkable. Often women just stick a pad on and carry on, thinking leaking while running is inevitable. It's really not, and you shouldn't put up with it.

Instead of giving up running, perhaps we need to think about thresholds, and adjust the duration or intensity of your run to take into account your pelvic floor's needs. If you can run for 20 minutes, or say, 3km, with no wet patch in your knickers, then stick with that time and no longer. Respect your boundaries and gently nudge them from time to time, but pay attention to your symptoms and adjust accordingly. Slower pace, shorter duration, whatever it takes to get to a symptom-free run. Notice how your pelvic floor feels in the days after your runs, and really take note of these and respond to what you're body is telling you. It's not forever, just for now, and it may change according to where you are in your cycle (see page 50).

Heavy lifting

This is a heavily debated aspect with regards to pelvic floor dysfunction, especially pelvic organ prolapse (POP). A case control study of 49 women with POP found that heavy occupational lifting was associated with POP.[15] A literature review also found that women undergoing surgery for POP were more likely to report a history of heavy occupational work.[16]

When we look at heavy lifting for exercise, one survey of over 3,900 women found physically active women who were lifting less than 15kg were more likely to report symptoms of POP than women lifting weight that was 50kg or more.[17]

They concluded that physically active women who lift heavy for exercise are not at an increased risk for POP. We can speculate that heavy lifting for work has an increased risk because of the amount of time spent lifting compared to a 1–2-hour workout a few times per week but as it stands there is simply not enough research to tell us if long-term exercise has a positive or negative effect on the pelvic floor.[18]

It has historically been recommended that people diagnosed with POP avoid lifting and high-impact activity. This can be devastating to people who are physically active. The diagnosis itself is a challenge and to then restrict an activity that has been a major part of their life is often what really takes the biggest toll on their mental health. Losing an activity that is meaningful to a person may also jeopardize the social aspect of fitness and may heighten feelings of being "broken" and alone or isolated.[19]

Fitness is an outlet for so many people and contributes to self-esteem, socialization, an uplifted mood and better body image. Losing their outlet can contribute to depression and decreased self-esteem.

Slowly the narrative and guidelines are shifting and people living with prolapse and incontinence can experience more freedom with their movement. If you are struggling with prolapse and are afraid to move, please know that you CAN lift, and you CAN run, and you CAN exercise if that is your goal. Working with a pelvic health physiotherapist and moving mindfully while respecting your symptoms will allow you to enjoy exercise and may even improve your pelvic floor function.

Stress

Stress is something we all face to varying degrees and for a variety of reasons. It is linked to a multitude of health conditions and can also contribute to pelvic floor challenges. When faced with a stressful situation, the sympathetic nervous system triggers the fight or flight response, which releases cortisol and puts us in a heightened state of awareness that may have us breathing faster, increased blood pressure and greater muscle tension, ready to flee the danger.

This tension can often be in the neck, the chest, the buttocks and the pelvis. There is a link between jaw tension (clenching the teeth which is a common reaction to stress), and tension in the hips and pelvis. It is common for midwives and doulas to coach their clients to relax their jaw by moaning or sighing during birth to help the pelvic floor release and allow the passage of the baby.[20]

During stressful situations the adrenal glands also release a hormone called adrenaline, which causes the body to divert blood flow away from the intestines and toward the brain, heart and lungs. This slows down intestinal movements, which may lead to constipation.

Meditation continues to be one of the top recommendations for stress reduction. There are many different forms but even ten minutes of quiet undisturbed time each day can help. For those who find sitting still hard and perhaps even stressful, consider yoga or a walk. Moving meditation has benefits as well. The key is to disconnect from work, your phone, kids, traffic – whatever stressors you deal with – and just breathe.

BOX BREATHING FOR RELAXATION

Box breathing is an option to practise if you begin to feel stressed, and build into a habit as soon as you feel stress within your body.

Imagine a box: you can trace the box this exercise is in. With each of the four sides, there is a breathing instruction.

- Inhale for a count of 4 along the top of the box.
- Hold your breath for a count of 4 down the side
- Exhale for a count of 4 along the bottom of the box
- Hold your breath for a count of 4 before beginning the box inhale again.

Something I recommend everyone do is walk ... every day, 3–5km if possible and in nature if you are fortunate enough to have some forest and trails nearby. Not only does walking reduce stress but it benefits your heart, your lungs, your brain and your pelvic floor too!

Toilet habits

How we go to the toilet, as well as how often we go, can influence our pelvic floor and our elimination, specifically constipation. We addressed constipation in the last section but will further address it here because it is so important!

"Normal" pooing habits are considered to be three times a day to three times a week, depending on what is usual for each individual. See the Rome criteria on constipation (details in the Resources). Constipation is defined as having fewer than three bowel movements per week. However, there are many who suggest that if you are not pooping once a day within the first hour of waking that you are constipated. It is typically characterized by hard lumpy stool or small pellet poos that are difficult to pass. Persistent constipation can affect the pelvic floor muscles and ligaments, as well as potentially exacerbating pelvic floor weakness and nerve damage. Constipation can also contribute to pressure on the bladder and urethra, which may cause increased frequency or urgency.

Constipation is very common and has consequences for the pelvic floor due to the risk of repetitive straining. The downward pressure from straining can contribute to organ prolapse, haemorrhoids, fissures and rectal prolapse. Preventing constipation is especially important if you already have any of these conditions. Rectoceles (page 34) add an additional challenge due to the fact that stool can get trapped in the bulge of the rectocele and make elimination more difficult, which can in turn lead to straining. Optimizing digestion and staying hydrated are essential for managing your pelvic health and avoiding constipation. Aim to drink 1.5–2 litres of fluid per day and approximately 35 grams of fibre, both soluble and insoluble. Working with a holistic nutritionist or dietician can be helpful as well.

As mentioned earlier, diet, hydration and stress reduction are key with regards to managing and eliminating constipation. Exercise is important to help literally keep things moving. Listening to your digestive signals is also vital and often when we are stressed or busy rushing around, we ignore signals, or *are not aware of the signals* to poo. When these signals are ignored, the stool will dry up, making them even more difficult to pass. If recommended by a pelvic health physio, using a laxative may be an option. Ideally this should not happen often because you can become dependent on stool stimulants or softeners, but for times like travelling, which can mess up your pooing routine, a stool softener and/or laxative can help prevent straining during the next bowel movement.

Posture on the toilet is also key. The "squatty potty" is a stool (no pun intended) that wraps around the base of your toilet and provides an elevated platform for your feet. This raises your knees above your hips and allows relaxation of a pelvic floor muscle called the puborectalis. It essentially takes the kink out of the rectum to allow stool to evacuate more easily. The squatty potty also has a slight forward angle that puts the feet into plantar flexion (toes pointing downwards), which can help relax the pelvic floor. It also helps to relax the jaw and mouth.

There's no need to buy a special device though: you can create your own squatty potty by using a toddler step/foot stool and placing your feet on it while you're on the toilet, to lessen the angle of your hips. Even better, slightly lean forward with your elbows resting on your knees, to lengthen your lumbar spine which allows a straighter "exit route" for your stool and means you won't need to strain.

A key point to remember is to not ignore the urge to poo. On the flipside, don't try to force a bowel movement if you don't feel the urge. Once you *do* feel the urge, sit down, elevate your feet on the stool and breathe deeply. It may help to rotate your torso from left to right, or even hold a rolled-up towel against your abdomen to help increase intra-abdominal pressure.

If nothing happens after five minutes, stand up. You can also try drinking a glass of lemon water, going for a walk or sitting on your heels in a kneeling position to see if that stimulates an urge. The best time to try to go is in the morning, 20 minutes after breakfast and a hot drink. Coffee has a stimulant effect on the bowel and possibly lemon. Get into a good habit of going every morning if you are very troubled with constipation – having a glass of lemon water, perhaps warmed, every morning can help stimulate digestion. Set your alarm a bit earlier to allow yourself quiet time to sit and sip, and wait to poo.

CHAPTER 4

PREGNANCY, BIRTH AND PELVIC FLOOR RECOVERY

Pregnancy, birth and motherhood provide such a fundamental "moment" in pelvic floor health that they deserve a chapter to themselves. It is arguable that if the male pelvic floor experienced trauma as early in life as the female pelvic floor, perhaps pelvic floor dysfunction would have received more investigation and respect from medical research and treatment options. As it is, too many young women are suffering from pelvic floor dysfunction, and without information and guidance, continue to do so into their menopausal years and old age. We need to halt this trend by empowering ourselves with information and knowledge earlier in life.

It is well documented and accepted that pregnancy and childbirth are risk factors for pelvic floor dysfunction. A 2003 study found that between 20% and 60% of pregnant women and one third of new mothers will experience stress urinary incontinence. In the last trimester, 48% of first-time mothers will experience incontinence and that goes up to 85% for women who have had multiple pregnancies.[1]

For women with urinary incontinence at 12 weeks postnatal, 92% of them would still have it five years later.[2] Another study showed that approximately three quarters of women who had urinary incontinence at three months postpartum still have it at six years postpartum.[3]

An interesting study looked at the responses of 482 women who were sent a survey to explore problems experienced by women one year after childbirth. It found the following:

- 87% of women experienced some type of perineal problem.
- 53.8% had some degree of stress incontinence and 36.6% had some degree of urge incontinence.
- 54.5% of women reported some type of sexual problem.
- 9.9% reported some degree of liquid faecal incontinence.
- 32.6% of women who had an episiotomy or tear still had some degree of pain.
- Problems are more common among women who had episiotomies or first- or second-degree tears (there were not enough women with third- or fourth-degree tears to allow an analysis of tear severity and perineal problems).
- 34.8% of women without perineal tears experienced stress incontinence versus 52.7% of women with a tear or episiotomy.
- 19.5% of women without perineal tears experienced urge incontinence, versus 29.2% of women with a tear and 38% of women with episiotomy.

Some interesting points were that women without tears or episiotomy still report stress incontinence, which suggests that it is not just those with perineal trauma who are at risk of pelvic floor dysfunction. It was also interesting to note that there was very little difference in stress incontinence rates between women who had an episiotomy and those who tore (grade 1 or 2). There has been a general trend away from performing routine episiotomies over the past few years.[4]

It is also becoming increasingly common for women to start their families later in life, which can increase the risk of developing incontinence. One study found that the prevalence of stress urinary incontinence 1–2 years after a vaginal birth was four times more common among women who were over 36 when they gave birth, compared to women under age 29. The older women who experienced stress incontinence during pregnancy were more likely to experience persistent symptoms, compared to those who had no stress incontinence in pregnancy.[5]

There is such a huge opportunity to educate pregnant women about their pelvic floor so they can make informed choices in their pregnancy fitness, their birth and their postpartum recovery. Recovering from pregnancy and birth really can be positively affected by your body awareness during pregnancy. Pregnancy used to be considered an ailment of sorts. Women were advised to rest and not do much. The pendulum started to swing and recently it has become the norm to celebrate extremes in pregnancy, and applaud those who are back to the gym at two weeks postpartum. In our social media driven world, people flaunt their beautiful bellies and compare the baby's size to fruits and vegetables in their daily posts. Once the baby is born, the post-birth belly becomes a place of shame and there is a race to *not* look pregnant as fast as possible. This takes a toll on the body, mentally and physically. The birth of a baby is significant – and equally so is the transition to motherhood. An emphasis on supporting the new mother in the early weeks postpartum is a necessary shift in the hopes of improving pelvic health outcomes for birthing people.

Pelvic floor exercises in pregnancy

It is so important to learn and practise pelvic floor exercises in pregnancy, if not sooner, and I offer a slight modification in the last few weeks of pregnancy. Typically people start their perineal massage around 35–37 weeks and I recommend a small change to performing kegels at this time. The inhales remain focused on the expansion of the ribs, the belly and the pelvic floor, and the exhales shift from contract and lift to keeping space and softening. In a vaginal birth, the second stage of labour, the push phase, is accompanied by exhaling. Normally we train the pelvic floor to engage on the exhale, but when giving birth it would be counterproductive to contract and lift the space we are trying to keep open to allow our baby to pass through.

So in the final weeks of pregnancy, I encourage practising an inhale to expand and imagine blossoming the vulva, then practise exhaling while maintaining that expansion. Simply blossom the vulva on the inhale and then practise exhaling while keeping their flower in bloom.

I then recommend this practice is taken into labour. Inhale to expand as they feel a contraction building then exhale through pursed lips while keeping the pelvic floor open and free.

In pregnancy and the early postpartum weeks, I do have a few "avoid" exercises that take into consideration the biomechanical changes that are happening, as well as the purpose of an exercise. I view birth as an event to be trained for and I promote movements that mimic labour and birth while also building a strong body for the challenges of parenthood. An exercise such as the plank is a static exercise, and is one that I don't recommend. It puts additional strain on the linea alba that is already stretching from the growing baby. If there are some potential negatives to an exercise that is not preparing the body to birth more powerfully, then I don't believe it is a useful thing to do.

Before the birth, there are many other changes happening during pregnancy that influence the inner core unit. Some of these are listed below:

Hormones in pregnancy

It is no secret that hormones play significant roles in pregnancy. The main ones that can affect the body most profoundly are:

Human chorionic gonadotropin (HCG)

This is the hormone that is secreted in your urine and is what the home pregnancy tests use to determine if you are pregnant or not. The role of HCG is to tell your body that there is a life form in your womb that needs to be nurtured as opposed to expelled. HCG also tells the ovaries to stop maturing an egg every month. This hormone is also responsible for increasing the blood supply to the pelvis which can contribute to an increase in the frequency of the bladder signaling to empty.

This increase in bladder signals can start to contribute to more frequent bathroom visits but it is important to recognize that it is not always because your bladder is full. A bladder should signal to empty every 2.5–4 hours. In pregnancy there is HCG, there is reduced space as the baby grows and therefore more pressure on the bladder which means you feel you need to empty it more often. This can in turn "train" the bladder to signal before it is completely full even after you are no longer pregnant. Once your baby is born, ensure you remember the 2.5–4-hour window and work to retrain your bladder.

Progesterone

Progesterone keeps the uterus muscle relaxed and inhibits it from contracting. Progesterone also relaxes all smooth muscle in the body which is important with regards to the sphincter muscles in the pelvic floor. It may contribute to constipation by relaxing the muscles associated with peristalsis in the intestines.

Constipation is common especially in early pregnancy. It is uncomfortable and can lead to straining, which can affect the pelvic floor. The pelvic floor will undergo a lot of strain during childbirth so you don't want to be adding more strain with your daily bowel movement. Ensure you stay well hydrated and eat high-fibre foods (both soluble and non-soluble fibre) to help make your bowel movements easy to pass. A footstool is also an essential tool to use not only for elimination purposes but also for keeping your body squat-ready. Squatting is very effective for labour as it increases the space of the pelvic outlet. A fun little sidebar here, the Squatty Potty could also be used as a birth stool if you don't have one at home or if the hospital you are birthing in doesn't have one.

Exercise and movement can also help with constipation so ensure you get out for a daily walk. Walking is also beneficial for the pelvic floor and, of course, mental wellbeing.

Oestrogen

Oestrogen stimulates hormone production in the fetus's adrenal gland and enhances your uterus, so it can respond to oxytocin when it is time to birth your baby. During the second trimester, oestrogen plays a major role in the development of the milk ducts, which in turn enlarges the breasts.

Growing breasts can influence your posture. The shoulders often round with the heaviness of fuller breasts, and you may start to lean back to counteract the shifting centre of gravity from your growing belly. A well-fitting maternity bra is essential, as is the awareness of how your body is adapting.

Relaxin

Relaxin is believed to be primarily responsible for relaxing the ligaments that support the joints and is often blamed for the aches and pains commonly associated with pregnancy. Relaxin is produced by the ovaries and the placenta and is responsible for relaxing the ligaments in the pelvis, as well as softening and lengthening the cervix. Relaxin is at its highest in the first trimester and at birth. It is not known exactly how long relaxin levels stay elevated in the body after the baby is born but it is estimated to be between four and nine months. You may feel less stable in all your joints, and particularly in your pelvis.

The linea alba (LA) is another area of the body that is influenced by relaxin. The LA is the connective tissue between the rectus abdominis muscles (more on this in Diastasis rectus abdominis, page 77). As the uterus grows, the linea alba must expand to accommodate it causing the rectus to move away from the midline (diastasis rectus abdominis).

Moving with awareness in pregnancy is essential. With the knowledge of how hormones are influencing your structures, understanding that your pelvis is less stable and that your abs are stretching beyond their optimal length, you can make appropriate exercise choices that safeguard and build your body, rather than put it at increased risk for injury and pelvic floor challenges.

Breathing

Early on in pregnancy hormones can contribute to a breathless feeling. Even though you are actually getting MORE oxygen into your system, it may not feel like it! As the pregnancy progresses and the baby grows, the space for the diaphragm to descend is reduced, which can make it difficult to take a deep breath. This can also be a way that non-optimal breathing patterns begin, especially if the body is compensating for the stretching of the outer abdomen by over-using or gripping the obliques.

Ensure you stand and move frequently through the day. Make time for stretching and release work for the side body and obliques, because when tension is held in the ribcage or the obliques it can restrict the expansion of the ribs and therefore the descent of the diaphragm during inhalation.

Alignment

The growth of the abdomen in pregnancy causes shifts in the centre of gravity. When not pregnant, your pelvis should be over your heels meaning the weight should be mainly in your heels and midfoot, not your forefeet, and your ribs should be over your pelvis. Some people claim that their feet "grow" in pregnancy, but it may be more accurately a result of weakness in the lateral hip rotators that causes the thighs to internally rotate, which then causes the arches of the feet to lower. Hormones may also contribute to the ligamentous arch in the foot softening, which can create the illusion that the foot is longer. Choosing exercise and movements that work on strengthening the lateral rotators of the hip will help, as will spending more time barefoot so that the muscles in the foot work as they should, rather than being restricted by the shoes.

As your belly grows you should still be able to keep your weight over your pelvis. Unfortunately, with the increased sitting we do these days and because of the lack of walking and squatting we do, our backsides typically don't have the mass or strength to counterbalance the growing belly. This results in compensations like tight hamstrings, a pelvis pushed forward, flat buttocks, and pelvic floor muscles that are short and tight. Glute work is especially important in pregnancy.

To find optimal alignment (while pregnant or not), stand with your feet hip-width apart and pointing forward. Back your pelvis up so that your perineum (the area between your vagina and anus) is over the space between your ankles. Now release your buttocks (I like to imagine blossoming, like a flower). Once you find better alignment it may feel unfamiliar. Many feel like they are going to tip forward or that they are sticking their bottom out. Better alignment is often quite a departure from where you normally are, so of course it will feel different and slightly unfamiliar. It is important to remember that alignment is the by-product. Constantly placing your ribs over pelvis and pelvis over ankles and relaxing your bum, especially while moving, is not realistic. As you build your awareness, spend less time sitting, and work on softening the muscles that are tight, so better alignment will just happen.

The abdomen

The abdominal wall is one part of the body that undergoes a lot of change and contributes to the shifting in the centre of gravity. With the pull of the growing belly, the tendency is for the pelvis to start to tip anteriorly, resulting in a more significant curve in the lumbar spine. As the pregnancy progresses, the natural reaction to the increased heaviness in front is to lean back and push the pelvis forward. This can contribute to a loss of the lumbar curve and glutes that no longer fire as they should. Many people are not aware of these subtle shifts occurring and think the resulting aches and pains are a normal part of pregnancy. The key is to be aware of your posture, release tension in the pelvic floor and ensure you work on building the glutes throughout pregnancy. This will result in less strain on the abdominal wall and less change in the centre of gravity.

In pregnancy, the abdomen faces significant stretch to the muscles and to the connective tissue – namely the linea alba – which contributes to diastasis recti (see below). While the condition is a normal adaptation to pregnancy, and we can't "prevent" it, you can definitely lessen its impact on the body. So it's a good idea to maintain your awareness of your Core Four activation while pregnant, and also participate in restorative exercise postpartum with the aim of reestablishing connective tissue integrity and tone in the muscles of the abdomen. More than 50% of women with diastasis recti have some form of pelvic floor dysfunction such as incontinence or prolapse.[6]

Diastasis rectus abdominis

By definition, diastasis rectus abdominis (or diastasis recti) is the separation of the right and left rectus abdominis muscles from the midline. The midline being the linea alba. Linea alba means "white line" and is the band of connective tissue that holds the rectus muscles in place at the midline of the abdomen. In pregnancy, that line can darken and it's termed linea nigra.

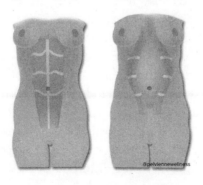

The linea alba is a complex connective tissue with lots of interwoven collagenous fibres. It's a central insertion point for the external obliques, the internal obliques and the transversus abdominis. The width of the linea alba or the distance between the left and right rectus muscles is referred to as the inter-recti distance (IRD). The IRD (or "gap" as many refer to it as) varies along its length from the xyphoid process to the pubic symphysis.

In terms of function, the linea alba plays a role in support and force distribution in our core. It's responsible for mechanical stability, and it helps maintain the abdominal muscles that are a certain proximity to each other. We don't know exactly what is normal for a given person. We do know that the linea alba softens during pregnancy to allow the two rectus bellies to curve and create space for the baby. The same could be said though for somebody, male or female, who is carrying more weight or girth in the abdomen.

The term "diastasis" means separation, but it can be misleading because there is *always* a gap between the rectus muscles – they are never fused together – and it has never been fully determined what a "normal" gap size is. This can mean people who find out they have diastasis recti after pregnancy, perhaps from a Pilates trainer or pelvic health physio, may have actually had that same size gap before pregnancy. One study noted that different normative values for IRD were found at different locations of the abdominal wall. In women who've had children, the IRD may be considered "normal" up to values wider than in those who haven't.[7]

More current research is recognizing that it is not really about the gap but rather the integrity of the connective tissue at rest and during movement – i.e. *does it activate when it should?* Diane Lee and Paul Hodges found in their study that when participants did the curl-up task, the IRD lessened but the connective tissue sagged or became distorted – meaning it lacked tension. Pre-activation of the TvA lessened the reduction of the IRD and reduced the distortion of the linea alba. They suggest that as the TvA tensions, it pulls the left and right rectus further apart, but the tension is what is needed to transfer loads/forces through the trunk effectively.[8]

Another study looking at linea alba distortion and stiffness found that DRA was associated with low linea alba stiffness and distortion during a semi curl-up task. Much of the early exercise prescription for diastasis was focused on the TvA, which we know plays a role, but it is becoming clear with more current research that a global approach that includes the entire abdominal wall may be most beneficial for the healing and management of diastasis recti.

If you've heard or read anything about diastasis, you've typically seen the "finger assessment", which is still used and can provide some meaningful information, when done correctly. It is a measurement tool that initially considered only the gap. But it has more recently been expanded to assess not only the gap but also the integrity of the connective tissue at rest, with a pelvic floor contraction, and in a variety of positions. So it's not a question of "closing the gap" but firing up the connection.

Whether or not DRA is a concern from a core function perspective lies more in the ability of a person to create and maintain tension in the connective tissue than on the distance between their two rectus muscles. A key component to generating and maintaining tension in the connective tissue is the pelvic floor. When the pelvic floor contracts, there is (or should be) a co-contraction of the transversus abdominis that tenses the connective tissue.

A lot of the information in social media focuses on the visual or aesthetic perspective of diastasis and promotes "closing the gap". While the gap is not *irrelevant*, the focus really should be on function first. Left untreated, or by focusing just on closing the gap, diastasis can lead to back pain, pelvic pain, incontinence, prolapse, increased risk of injury in the abdomen, and a non-active abdominal wall.

The generally accepted approach to help heal and manage it is to address posture and breathing, establish a connection between the brain and the pelvic floor in a lying or seated position, and then gradually load the connective tissue and challenge the muscles. Gradual loading of the connective tissue is key, and is done by varying the positions for pelvic floor exercise. Once the pelvis is functioning well, with tension being generated and maintained in a variety of positions, then it is time to progress to more intense exercises such as planks, push-ups and rotation movements that load not only the connective tissue but also the muscles.

The impact of birth on the body

On top of all of the changes and adaptations that are happening in the pregnant body, there is the birth itself. Childbirth is very closely tied to pelvic floor injury and lingering dysfunction, both vaginal and caesarean birth. In a vaginal birth, and caesarean where you have laboured first, there is significant stretch and pressure on the nerves, tissue, and the muscles in the pelvic floor. People who experience third- and fourth-degree tears are at greater risk of challenges, especially persistent pain and anal incontinence. OASIS (obstetric anal sphincter injuries) include third- and fourth-degree tears. Of the 85% of women who tear during childbirth[9] 0.6%–11% will experience a 3rd or 4th degree tear.[10] More awareness is being created for women who have suffered a birth injury by organizations such as Masic in the UK, whose aims are to raise public awareness and help injured women, support research and prevention and educate medical professionals.

A group of multi-disciplinary professionals in Canada has similar goals of informing medical professionals, providing resources to injured mothers and campaigning for prevention in prenatal education.

The most common long-term challenges people with OASIS face are pain with sex, perineal pain and anal incontinence.[11] OASIS is a main reason for delayed intercourse after birth and for pain with sex at one year postpartum; however, between 60%

and 80% of women are asymptomatic 12 months postpartum ,following an external anal sphincter repair.

How pushing affects the pelvic floor

Pushing time also needs to be considered. It is generally accepted that a second-stage labour (the push phase) lasting about an hour or less would be ideal, with two hours being the max. There are however many people who push for three, four or five hours which can be physically exhausting, contribute to significant swelling in the perineum and actually increase the likelihood of tearing. A 2009 study reported that first-time mums who push for over two hours and second-time moms who push for more than one hour are more likely to have third- and fourth-degree tears.[12]

Really short push times are not always ideal either. When things progress very quickly, the tissues of the pelvic floor do not have time to slowly stretch and accommodate the baby's head, which can sometimes contribute to greater risk of tearing. Long push times mean more time that the muscles are under the stretch, compression and pressure which could contribute to increased risk of nerve degeneration, loss of tissue integrity, and muscle control.

Episiotomy surgery and the pelvic floor

An episiotomy is a surgical cut in the perineum, made to create more space for baby to be birthed. Episiotomies are performed less often as standard procedure than they used to be, as it has become clear they may contribute to more pain and healing difficulties postnatally. They may not be performed routinely, but they do still happen – so it is a good idea to ask your hospital policy/midwife/care provider if appropriate, if episiotomy is a routine procedure – and if it is, make sure you do your research and make a conscious choice – remember *you do have a choice*. You can outline in your birth preferences that you would rather avoid an episiotomy.

Perineal massage is often promoted as a way to prevent tearing, and some research supports this. It is typically done between 35–37 weeks of pregnancy. It can also be performed during labour, but in my opinion this is not ideal. It can contribute to greater swelling in the tissues, which can increase the risk of tearing. It is also invasive. Labour and birth is a time to leave the birthing person be, she needs support but not *interruption*; sometimes the act of stretching the tissues can create a distraction that takes the person "out of the zone". Instead, a warm compress held on the perineum can be soothing and can also allow the midwife or doula to apply counter pressure on the perineum as the baby's head is crowning. Ask your midwife about this in your antenatal checks. You want to know the practices of your midwife BEFORE you are in labour.

Birthing positions

Something else to consider in advance is what birth positions are most optimal in terms of facilitating birth and protecting the pelvic floor. It is beneficial to talk to your midwife and/or doula about your position options in one of your antenatal appointments. It has been shown that the lithotomy position can be less advantageous for the birthing person however it is still the most common position used. The lithotomy position is a back lying position and can be associated with a longer pushing time. There is often more pressure and strain on the nerves and muscles. The back-lying position and even the semi-reclined position lock the sacrum in place. The sacrum should ideally be unobstructed so it can move as needed, as baby moves into and out of the pelvis. When the sacrum is locked in place it narrows the pelvic outlet, and also does not allow for the tailbone to get out of the way, which can both contribute to more difficulty for the person pushing. Birthing in a side-lying position has been shown to be the most likely to preserve the perineum, meaning less likelihood of tearing. There are many antenatal education programmes that provide essential labour prep info, such as hypnobirthing. Find one that covers the biomechanical changes of pregnancy, dynamic birth position options and information about postpartum recovery.

Nothing guarantees there will be no tearing but when you're informed, have trained your body for optimal birth positions and have a midwife or clinician that supports your wishes, it can reduce the chances of perineal tears and of interventions such as ventouse and forceps. Of the women who have a forceps-assisted birth, 50% may experience after-effects in their pelvic floor function and sensation.[13]

Third- and fourth-degree tears are common with a forceps-assisted birth and so it may be considered potentially more challenging in terms of recovery as well. Vaginal birth with forceps is a leading risk factor for levator ani avulsion (LAA), the detachment of the puborectalis muscle (one of the pelvic floor muscles) from its attachment on the pubis. It can be partial or complete and in some minor cases it may resolve on its own over time.[14] People with LAA are at greater risk for developing POP[15] and are more likely to experience POP recurrence after corrective surgery.

Abdominal birth (caesarean section)

What about abdominal birth? Is the pelvic floor protected by having a caesarean (c-section)? While having a caesarean can produce a protective effect against some pelvic floor challenges, it does not eliminate the possibility of developing incontinence, POP or other challenges. It's important to know that pregnancy itself causes immense pressure on the pelvic floor even before the birth itself. Many people believe that if they have a caesarean, they are immune to pelvic floor challenges. The unhelpful phrase "too posh to push" suggests that caesarean is an "easy option" – which makes us forget that it's major surgery.

People may elect to have a caesarean for myriad factors: for health reasons; due to baby's breech or transverse position; maybe they have an existing POP and want to avoid further damage; or have experienced previous birth trauma. Others may go through labour and maybe even push, and then end up having an unplanned caesarean birth. As discussed earlier, there are a lot of adaptations and influences on the pregnant body before birth that can contribute to the development of pelvic floor dysfunction.

Caesarean section is *major abdominal surgery*. Several layers of skin, fat and connective tissue, and the womb itself, are cut through and then sewn back up with different layers of sutures – so a lot of the healing and scar tissue will not be seen. The natural balance of these layers is therefore altered, and this can lead to changes in sensation and loss of nerve endings, sometimes cause issues with being able to connect to your pelvic floor, and its function. Abdominal surgery also inherently disrupts the regular balance of your abdomen, and of the diaphragm's movement within your torso, and this can have a huge effect on your pelvic floor efficacy and function. It takes conscious effort to reconnect and repair, to rebuild the full circuit to work again.

Abdominal and scar massage

Abdominal massage is a vital part of any postnatal healing toolkit, whether belly birth or vaginal birth, to release tension in the space between the diaphragm and pelvic floor to unlock optimum function.

Scar massage, where the scar itself and the area around the scar is gently palpated and moved around, may help prevent adhesions forming (areas of connective tissue which can become sticky like Velcro after surgery, and can "glue" organs together or otherwise impede movement and muscular function). It is suitable from six weeks after caesarean – but also useful even years after birth, and can help to stimulate circulation to the area, reduce swelling and enhance sensation as well. It's an important body-management practice that can be done by yourself or by a massage therapist or pelvic health physio, to reduce the build up of scar tissue and formation of adhesions. Regular abdominal massage is a way to enable the abdominal organs to reassemble to their pre-pregnancy position after pregnancy and the disruption of surgery, and this enhances optimal pelvic floor function.

Pelvic floor massage post-birth

We know about perineal massage before birth: what is less widely heard of as massage being a part of the postnatal healing toolkit. Gentle touch from when your wound has healed, and as long as you can do so without pain, can help to break down scar tissue, and reduce swelling, stimulate blood flow to the area and help rebuild sensation. There's no need to necessarily use a massage oil, but there are some special "vagina oils" available

The mother's rebirth

Childbirth is an epic, transformative event in a person's life. Emotionally, physically, mentally, spiritually … every element is brought into birth and so many new parents feel at their weakest after participating in one of the most amazing feats of strength. They are so attracted to and influenced by images and messaging around being strong and "getting their body back" that they forget to celebrate how amazing they are and how incredible the body is. There is a rush to not look pregnant any more, and little to no attention is paid to healing and recovery. Women feel like they need to be supermums, and may not have thought about postpartum support – or may have turned it down fearing it would be a sign of weakness. New parents want to *feel like themselves* again. To get back to "normal" activities. Lose the baby weight. To get back to working out. Mums are often attracted to the activities that are hard and intense because they feel that it is what they need to do in order to feel strong and reach their goal weight. This mentality is not serving new mums at all, and perhaps it is the rise in intense activity, coupled perhaps with a more sedentary slow-paced lifestyle with a baby that is contributing to pelvic floor dysfunction.

Once the baby is born, there is a period of time when I recommend avoiding certain movements to give the body time to heal and to ensure the core has been retrained. I do recommend avoiding things like planks along with high-impact activities initially, favouring core-connection activities like core breath with bridge (see page 135) and squats (see page 138).

I have a saying … "Mummy and bootcamp do not belong in the same sentence." You can absolutely return to bootcamp, or run, or do CrossFit, but those activities should not be what you choose in order to "get your body back". Honour your body, the need to recover and the need for a gradual return to fitness. More and more professionals agree that it can take upward of a year postpartum to fully recover and it is important to remember that once postpartum, always postpartum. The body has changed. The landscape is different. What you did before may not be what your body needs after pregnancy and that's okay. Be curious and aware. Listen to what your body needs and seek the help of professionals who can help you navigate the amazing options for movement you have.

Postnatal depression and pelvic floor dysfunction

Pelvic floor dysfunction can be associated with trauma, which may in turn heighten mental health struggles. When considering postnatal depression (PND), it is not surprising to find that women struggling with PND are also experiencing pelvic floor challenges. A retrospective chart review was performed of 294 women referred to a specialty postpartum perineal clinic and it was found that "Urinary incontinence during and after pregnancy and referral for pain were pelvic floor symptoms independently associated with a positive postpartum depression screen in women referred to a specialty perineal clinic. Therefore, consideration should be given to depression screening in women presenting with perinatal urinary incontinence and persistent postpartum pain, as these women may be at increased risk of developing postpartum depression."[16]

There are many conservative options for treating pelvic floor dysfunction as well as surgical options. Both seem to play a role in improving mental health. One study showed that depression and quality of life improved in all patients after three months of pessary use.

Another study investigating surgical outcomes for POP found that quality of life and depression dramatically improved following surgical treatment. The important thing for people to know is that there are many options, and a big part of coping with pelvic floor dysfunction is a supportive healthcare team that can help you navigate the options and ensure you are making informed choices in both conservative and surgical options.

There exists an incredible opportunity to educate people while they are pregnant so they can make informed decisions in their pregnancy, birth and postpartum recovery. In France, all pregnant women and new mothers are referred to pelvic floor physiotherapy that is paid for by the government. This is often seen as the Holy Grail, and highlighted as something we should all aspire to – it's worth noting that there is mixed evidence from France, with some studies showing it makes no difference in pelvic floor dysfunction rates in the long term. This shows the human flaw in pelvic flaws: taking action and responsibility for your own healing is the most important aspect of your healing journey. Pelvic floor health requires ongoing maintenance, commitment and attention, *for life*. Comprehensive screening postnatally may the best option. Imagine if all birthing women were educated about pelvic health before they were faced with this challenge, and supported adequately afterward?

For now, people need to advocate for themselves, often relying on medical information on social media and online research, which can be very overwhelming and often sends people further into depression. Thankfully, more and more fitness and wellness professionals are becoming educated and referring to pelvic health physiotherapy. Social media can be a fantastic place for people to learn and connect with others going through similar struggles. It is gradually becoming more acceptable to talk about incontinence without shame or just laughing it off.

A lot of people follow me or coach with me because they know I have experience of prolapse. They see me exercise, and that can be a source of inspiration. Many people are told they can't lift, or run, or exercise intensely any more. Seeing someone else doing it while managing a prolapse helps give them hope, shows them they are not alone and that help exists, and this can often be the key to healing both physically and mentally. Make sure you curate your social media carefully, from sources who share evidence-based reputable physio-led information, rather than perhaps some of those who may be focusing more on aesthetics.

Postpartum recovery

The pelvic floor takes a minimum of four to six months to heal after pregnancy and can even be upward of a year. There were nine months of changes and adaptations and then there was the birth – vaginal or surgical. It doesn't make sense to assume that at six weeks after giving birth, all of your body's adaptations have vanished and the body has returned to its pre-pregnancy state. The postpartum body needs time to rest and recover, and then retrain the core synergy that may have been affected or lost in pregnancy and birth.

The first 40 days

Many cultures around the world honour the first 40 days post birth and believe they set the new mother up for the next 40 years. Healing practices such as warming massages, belly wrapping and eating warm nourishing foods like bone broths, soups and stews, are all part of a philosophy known as Mother Roasting or Mother Warming. The belief is that the body has "opened" in pregnancy and birth and is prone to "wind" or cold. Wrapping, massages, rest, baths and foods are all used to help keep the body warm, support involution of the uterus, replenish lost chi and "close" the body. A fantastic book that explores the traditional practice deeper is *The First Forty Days* by Heng Ou.

Wrapping provides temporary external support to the pelvis and lower abdomen, where the muscles have stretched beyond their optimal length and are hindered in their ability to contribute to control. Wrapping is not waist training and is like a gentle hug to the pelvis instead of a waist-cinching measure. I view it as swaddling for the new mum. While not an evidence-based recommendation: just as swaddling a new baby can be comforting and help them feel safe, wrapping the new mum can be supportive and provide security in movement in the early weeks postpartum. The other key factor is that wrapping alone is not enough. The inner core unit needs to be retrained, and the sooner the restorative exercises start, the better. Doing nothing at all (in terms of movement or pelvic floor awareness exercises) and then getting a six-week "green light" for exercise is not serving new mothers. Gentle walks, breathing practices and pelvic floor muscle training should be done before the six-week check in.

When you make your postnatal plan it's worth factoring in pelvic health physio as part of your "mother plan" alongside thinking about setting up the nursery and which buggy you're going to buy. Physical recovery after birth is much more needed than a bunch of cute baby clothes. In the UK, NHS referral is free, you just have to ask for it. Unfortunately for a lot of people physiotherapy is something that we need to pay for, and this means that pelvic health recovery becomes linked to economic status – which isn't right and why we need to spread awareness of the ways you *can* optimize your pelvic health with whatever means and sources of guidance are available to you.

Retraining your core

I recommend starting the pelvic floor or core breath (page 104) exercises in the first few days to help stimulate sensation, increase circulation to aid in healing, and activate muscle memory. Initiation of the pelvic floor muscle training in the immediate postpartum period may reduce the risk of future urinary incontinence.[17] Voluntarily contracting the pelvic floor muscles in the early days post-birth may be uncomfortable, especially if you have had any tearing or an episiotomy. I recommend doing a dedicated breathing practice where you visualize the expansion of the pelvic floor muscles on the inhale, and the contract and lift of the pelvic floor on the exhale. Just watch what is happening in your mind, as you breathe in and out – and then as soon as you are able, add in the voluntary pelvic floor activation on the exhale to support continued healing and retraining of your pelvic floor muscles.

The next exercise I recommend starting whenever you feel ready in the weeks post-birth is the bridge (page 135). Glutes are important as support for the pelvis. Bridges also offer a gentle inversion which may help realign the organs after the downward forces of childbirth. Lying on your back is also a low-load position to begin your early pelvic floor muscle training.

Next, I add in a seated weight-transfer exercise to help retrain pelvic control, squats, standing one-leg balances and lunges (see pages 137–39). These are all done with the core breath to retrain the Core Four synergy in movement, and by about eight weeks postpartum I have my clients start adding in exercises specific to what they want to go back to. The key is *gradual progression*. Even if my client has done the recovery protocol and seen a pelvic floor physiotherapist, they will not immediately go back to the weight they lifted before, or the same number of sets and reps, or intensity. They are still very much in the retraining phase for four to six months *at least*. Postpartum healing is not linear, and it's common to experience setbacks. We have to be gentle with ourselves.

Returning to running

Runners are a difficult group to hold back. I know, because I was one. I was desperate to run again after birthing. I tried a little jog at two weeks postpartum. DO NOT DO THIS! I quickly realized that it did not feel good, so I stopped. Looking back, I now cringe but there was simply no information available about return to exercise postpartum. Runners want to run, and in order to return to running successfully, a few milestones need to be met, like walking. We literally need to walk before we run, so a brisk 30-minute walk (symptom free and with optimal form) is a prerequisite for running. Single leg balance exercises are key – one-leg balance, single-leg squats, single-leg hops etc. Not all at once and not all right away. Gradual progression. I repeat … GRADUAL PROGRESSION.

Running and other high impact activity is associated with a sudden rise in intra-abdominal pressure that can be extra troublesome for the postpartum body. The importance of strength, speed and coordination of the pelvic floor muscles is essential to carry out their role of continence and organ support during high impact activities. High-impact exercise was found to have a 4.59-fold increased risk of pelvic floor dysfunction compared to low impact exercise. I have linked to the physio-authored *Return to Running Guidelines* in the Resources.

New mothers need time to heal, a progressive recovery exercise-based programme and targeted activities that are eventually loaded in order to retrain the strength, endurance and anticipatory elements of the core.

Pregnancy and childbirth takes your pelvic floor and core strength to its limits, but there are always ways you can strengthen and rebuild. Please don't ever accept any pelvic floor and core issues as "just part of being a mum", it's simply not the case. You are worthy of healing. Make this book your pocket cheerleader for honouring your pelvic floor healing for life.

CHAPTER 5

THE NON-PHYSICAL EFFECTS OF PELVIC FLOOR DYSFUNCTION

The affect on mental health

Awareness about pelvic health is growing; however, it is still very much a topic that is difficult for most to talk about, and information is focused mainly on the physical symptoms associated with challenges like incontinence and prolapse. There is another aspect to pelvic health that has rarely been addressed and that is the toll that it can have on our mental health.

A study of more than 100 women with pelvic floor dysfunction found a significant association between depression and pelvic floor dysfunction.[1] Women are often fed messages from media and incontinence pad manufacturers that it is "just part of being a woman", reducing it to an "oops! moment", and we're encouraged to believe that you can simply put a pad in and you magically get your confidence back. These same women have often been suffering in silence for years because they have felt ashamed or embarrassed and when they finally *do* seek help, they are dismissed by their doctor, which leaves them feeling even more hopeless.

Feelings of hopelessness, guilt and shame are very common with pelvic floor dysfunction, and often a cause of then starting to withdraw from social interactions, exercise and intimacy, which leads to feelings of isolation, and can contribute to relationship struggles as well.

Incontinence, particularly faecal incontinence, and pelvic organ prolapse can hugely interfere with quality of life and have a negative influence on body confidence and mental wellbeing. Both are laced with taboo and shame, and this silence often means negative feelings multiply. "I feel broken", "I should have stopped running when I was pregnant", "I wish someone had told me about this before". These are all comments and sentiments felt and shared by women who feel let down and resentful, as well as fearful about their quality of life going forward. Pelvic health is so intricately tied to all aspects of our life that it can feel overwhelming and discouraging to understand what it means for the future. Going to a pelvic health physio – pushing for referral by your doctor even if they seem sceptical – can help you answer questions, develop a long-term strategy to manage and improve symptoms, and help move from overwhelm to positivity and acceptance.

Reduce or avoid exercise

So much information about pelvic floor dysfunction and exercise recommends avoiding certain exercises. The "don't do" list is longer than the "do" list. I was part of this mindset early on in my work. Ten years ago there was very little research about diastasis and prolapse. These words were not even known in the fitness realm, and there was not yet the collaboration between physiotherapists and fitness professionals that exists today. We are all more informed now, partly because of research, partly because of experience and partly because of social media.

We know more because we have tried more, we have questioned more and we have learned more. Ten years ago I and many of my pelvic health colleagues (often referred to as the #pelvicmafia) were proceeding with caution with our clients and our own bodies. Movement was very restrictive.

Slowly but surely, people started to push the boundaries and refused to accept the limitations being suggested – no lifting, no twisting, no running, no jumping – how could it be that we needed to eliminate these movements from our life? I remember questioning this with my internal voice, but not having the courage to speak out. As the boundaries were pushed, opinions were shared and new research began.

The pendulum is now swinging back, and more and more physios and trainers are recognizing that every body is different. Even two people who have a stage-2 prolapse will have different movement capabilities. Restrictive "avoid" lists are becoming a thing of the past, and there is a move toward a more individualized approach. There are still many individuals who may not have worked with a pelvic health physiotherapist or a core-informed trainer who are limiting or avoiding exercise for fear of making their condition worse, but movement is essential not only for our pelvic health but also for our whole-body (and mind) health.

The key lies in finding the movement that you enjoy and that allows you to manage your symptoms. I often say to work out in your symptom-free zone: if you go for a run, check your knickers for dampness, and scale down your distance or intensity until you can run dry, for example. But I want to also highlight that symptoms can be helpful reminders that keep us in check. I would say most people want to be symptom free, myself included, but I have come to recognize that symptoms vary from day to day and are dependent on so many things. Symptoms are not an indication of severity or of things worsening … they are just symptoms and many things contribute to symptoms.

We can harness our symptoms as a guide to direct our movement. I choose to do more low-impact, restorative exercise on days when I am symptomatic, and I also track my cycle so I can plan ahead (see the Menstruation section in Chapter 3 for more). Exercise with body awareness and intuition, meaning choose to move each day in a way that supports your mental and physical wellbeing, energy levels and symptoms.

Relationships and intimacy

If you are struggling with incontinence or prolapse, you might withdraw from friends and intimacy with a partner – shame and embarrassment and simply the lack of it being a "conversational topic" become obstacles too difficult to deal with, and it can have a devastating impact on relationships.

A survey conducted by Netmums for the Chartered Society of Physiotherapy (CSP) and the Royal College of Midwives (RCM) showed that half of the women surveyed said *they had never spoken to anyone about their pelvic floor issues.*

- Only 31% said they had spoken to their husband or partner, while just 19% had discussed it with their mother, sister or other close relative.
- Six in ten felt the subject was "taboo" and 56% said they felt embarrassed about the problem, with 16% feeling ashamed about it.
- Most worryingly of all, three quarters of women said they had never sought help from a health professional for this *treatable condition.*

Many partnered women don't even tell their significant other what they are dealing with because they are ashamed or embarrassed, or don't want their partner to think they aren't sexy anymore.

Pelvic floor dysfunction can have a very negative impact on self-esteem and body confidence, and fear of "accidents" or a partner seeing, feeling or smelling something leads many to avoid intimacy all together. This withdrawal without an explanation can lead to the partner feeling they aren't loved, that the relationship is ending and they are uncertain about what to do. When the truth is shared, most partners feel a sense of relief and are keen to find ways to be supportive. Seeking the help of a couples or relationship or sexual wellness counsellor can be very helpful.

Please speak up. You're NOT alone. There are others out there. I have included lots of organizations and books in the Resources section which will provide support and solace.

Let's talk about sex, baby!

Sex is good for our whole-body health, but it is often not something that we bring up in our checks with our doctor. One study found that over 60% of doctors do not proactively address sexuality with patients. There are probably also many women who don't want to bring it up with their healthcare provider for fear of being judged, or maybe sometimes because they don't want the awkwardness, or even make their doctor feel uncomfortable. Don't allow embarrassment and silence to steal your sex life. Don't feel awkward or embarrassed – chances are, your doctor or physiotherapist has heard it all before! We need to talk about sex.

Sex is good for the pelvic floor – consider it a fun pelvic floor workout! But many women struggling with incontinence of any kind or pelvic organ prolapse or pain will often avoid partnered sexual activity and may even avoid self-pleasure. There is shame and embarrassment and often an inability to fully let go and be present in the moment. Thoughts like "can she/he feel it?", "do I smell?", "can they see it?", and the fear of wetting the bed – or worse. It is difficult to relax and "enjoy the moment" with these fears running through your head. The muscles are also in a tense state. Not wanting anything to leak out or organs to bulge means the pelvic floor muscles will be in an overactive state which is also not conducive to a positive sexual experience and may inhibit orgasm. The pelvic floor is designed to stretch during sex which can stimulate the muscles and nerves. When in a stressed or constricted state or where there is a loss of sensation, which is common in those with pelvic floor dysfunction, it can mean sex is less satisfying or possibly not even possible.

An orgasm is like a bunch of involuntary kegels and could be counted towards your daily pelvic floor exercise. Learning how to contract and relax your pelvic floor muscles and then building strength and endurance and suppleness that can in turn make your orgasms stronger and can improve your overall experience during sex (partnered or not).

Pelvic floor exercise, including sex, may actually contribute to an improvement in pelvic floor muscle function and even symptoms.

Sex encourages blood flow and circulation which can enhance arousal and lubrication. You can also use sex as an opportunity to practice your pelvic floor exercise. Kegels during arousal can also heighten the sensation and may help in achieving orgasm.

Painful sex

Pain with sex is another important factor to consider. There can be varying types of pain with dyspareunia being one of the more common. Childbirth is a risk factor for developing genito-pelvic pain and/or dyspareunia during the postpartum period and potentially in the longer term. Dyspareunia is defined as persistent or recurrent genital pain when sexual intercourse or other sexual activity that involves penetration is attempted or pain during these sexual activities. The pain may be superficial or deep and can result from vaginal dryness or disorders of the genital organs.

Another pain syndrome that can interfere with sex is vaginismus, which is when there is an involuntary tightening of the pelvic floor muscles that causes burning, pain and challenges with penetration. Primary vaginismus is associated with "first-time" intercourse where penetration seems physically impossible. Secondary vaginismus is when there was previous history of normal penetrative sex, however there is now an unexplained, ongoing tightness which can often be attributed to a negative or traumatic pelvic or sexual experience. Women who are avoiding sex because of incontinence or prolapse may develop patterns of gripping in the pelvic floor muscles, which could in turn contribute to secondary vaginismus.

Pelvic floor muscle training with a physiotherapist can be very beneficial in reducing symptoms. A lot of women feel that they have "got their sex life back" after working with a physio, their sensation is restored and sex is a completely new experience, and this can truly be transformational in terms of quality of life and general health.

CHAPTER 6

SOLUTIONS FOR MANAGING PELVIC FLOOR DYSFUNCTION

We've explored the many things that can go awry with your pelvic floor, and how to recognize what might be wrong, so hopefully you're feeling empowered to investigate what is up and take ownership of your pelvic floor health. Now we can go through the wealth of options you have to restoring your floor to even better than its former glory. The first port of call should always be a trip to your pelvic health physio. They will create a treatment programme for you. And beyond that, this chapter will outline the many other strategies you can try, to enhance your pelvic floor, and overall health and wellbeing.

Pelvic floor physiotherapy

Pelvic health physiotherapists have particular expertise and training in assessing and treating the pelvic floor. They will perform an internal assessment (through the vagina) to assess and treat conditions like incontinence, organ prolapse, pelvic pain, painful sex.

When you first see a physio, they will take a thorough health history with you and will typically do some form of physical assessment (not always internal) during your first session. They may look at your posture and assess your breathing, observe and check your pelvic floor engagement in different positions and with movement. The internal assessment is done only if you feel comfortable and provide full consent. They used gloved fingers to assess the external genitalia to screen for scarring and certain conditions. With your consent, they will then use one or two gloved fingers inserted into the vagina to assess overall tone and if the tone is balanced, meaning there should be an appropriate level of "give" when the muscles are palpated and gently stretched. They will also assess for prolapse. They will then monitor your ability to contract *and relax* your pelvic floor muscles.

Some therapists use an ultrasound machine to get a better picture or to use as biofeedback, which can be helpful for people who are lacking sensation. That being said, most like to rely on their hands as opposed to a machine. If they find any scar tissue that needs to be mobilized they will treat that and then give you some homework to do before your next session. Homework may include posture work, stretches, strengthening exercises, pelvic floor exercises and muscle training, good toilet habits and maybe even discuss how you could explore options with a nutritionist or counsellor if needed. How many sessions you need will depend on many things such as time, cost, status of your pelvic floor etc. A lot of women I see say, "Well, I get a smear test (pap) every 3 years". But a smear test is very different from a pelvic floor physio assessment. Smear tests (pap smears) are not designed to assess the pelvic floor – they are screening for cancer – which is incredibly important, but not useful for determining the function of the pelvic floor.

When I began selling the EPI-NO, pelvic health physiotherapists began referring people to me. To ensure I could best help their patients, I needed to learn more about what they did. Carolyn Vandyken is a pelvic health physiotherapist in Ontario, Canada and is the first physio I met. She sat with me for over an hour and taught me about some of the inner workings of the pelvic floor and about how PFPT's assess and treat patients. I was blown away to say the least. I came out of that meeting asking myself "How is it that MOST WOMEN, especially women who have been pregnant, ARE NOT seeing a pelvic floor physio in pregnancy and postnatally?" Pelvic floor physiotherapy is arguably the most underused women's health resource we have, and one that should not need to be an out-of-pocket expense.

I made it my mission that day to passionately promote pelvic floor physiotherapy, and improve awareness and *options* for people wanting or needing help with their pelvic health. I hope that one day it is government funded in all countries around the globe. To find a physio in your area, you can do an online search for "pelvic floor physical therapy" or "pelvic health physiotherapy" and your city. I have included useful websites in the Resources. In the UK there is a directory for NHS and private physios in pelvic health at www.squeezyapp.com/directory. Pelvic, Obstetric and Gynaecological Physiotherapy (POGP) is also a good place to search for practitioners. You can also check out the directory at pelvicguru.com, which is global and growing every day.

Seeing a pelvic health physiotherapist can be life-changing, and if you're hesitating about going – please don't, ask to be referred or book yourself an appointment today. In the UK, in 2018 the government announced that as part of the 10-year plan for the NHS all women would see a pelvic health physiotherapist as part of the standard pathway of care. We can change the world by supporting one another, spreading awareness and advocating for women's health to be higher on the agenda. I also hope to see more collaboration between the medical community, pelvic health physios and fitness professionals, as we truly benefit from a village.

Pelvic floor muscle training

The pelvic floor muscles benefit from training, just like the rest of the body – and just like the rest of the body, they need a balance between strength, endurance and flexibility. We have slow-twitch and fast-twitch fibres in the pelvic floor, and training these muscles with a blend of slow holds and quick contract/releases is essential. This type of pelvic floor muscle training is voluntary, meaning you are *making* the contractions and relaxations happen. Treatment from a pelvic health physiotherapist may include some or all of the following types of modalities: strengthening exercises – for example pelvic floor exercises (kegels), relaxation exercises, breath work, trigger point release, manual therapy, biofeedback, ultrasound, electrotherapy and lifestyle education.

Pelvic floor muscle training is not a quick fix. Pelvic floor fitness is very much a lifestyle commitment. It is something we always need to be aware of and working on as we age and move through various life events and stages. You can't "fix your pelvic floor for life" – it's ongoing maintenance, much like dental care. The type of pelvic floor muscle training a person needs will change and evolve with different phases of life. Pregnancy is an example of a specific life stage that will require a different type of training than a non-pregnant woman in menopause. Surgery, falls, car accidents, stress, trauma, hormones, new activities … these will all influence the needs of the pelvic floor.

Once you know the basics, you are well-armed to manage your pelvic health for life.

Pelvic floor exercises (Kegels)

Kegels are a form of pelvic floor muscle training. They involve a voluntary contract, lift and release of the muscles. As mentioned earlier, these exercises are often done incorrectly – many assume it's just a squeeze and forget about the lift, or more importantly, the letting go. Imagery is helpful when learning to recruit the pelvic floor muscles properly.

Research suggests that the best way of engaging your pelvic floor is as follows:

- Take a deep breath in to relax your belly.
- As you breathe out, draw in your back passage as if you're stopping passing wind.

- Travel that engagement forward towards the front, and lift up.
- Hold this engagement. Check that there is no tension anywhere in the buttocks, inner thighs, shoulders or jaw.
- Breathe in and fully release and relax the pelvic floor.

This may work for you, but you might find that other imagery works better – it is about which cue elicits the desired response.[1]

Popular cues for finding your pelvic floor

- Imagine sipping a thick smoothie through a straw with your vagina
- Imagine picking up a blueberry with your vagina and anus.
- To help with the release end of the engagement, imagine your pelvic floor like a jellyfish softly floating on the inhale and propelling upward during the exhale.

Seeing a pelvic health physiotherapist can help you determine which is *your* best cue. Some personal trainers can also use some specific assessments and movement screens to help you find the best cue.

You can also use a biofeedback device, or your own fingers. Insert one or two fingers into your vagina and then engage your pelvic floor. Do you feel a gentle hug of your fingers as well as a drawing up movement? Are you holding your breath? Did you inhale or exhale to do engage the pelvic floor? Now, can you let the hug and lift go? You can even use a mirror, and check your vulva for any sign of your movement. If you are engaging, you will see that your vagina "winks" at you.

If you have a partner, you can also ask your partner to use their fingers, or penis if your partner is male. Ask them what they feel, and allow them to coach you. A hug, a gentle lift and a letting go is what you are after. This takes the pelvic floor through the full range of motion.

THE PELVIC FLOOR AND BREATHING

The pelvic floor moves in synergy with the diaphragm. Remember the synergy of the Core Four (page 17)?

What happens when you breathe in?

- The in-breath draws air into the body
- The ribs expand to allow space for the lungs to fill with air.
- The belly expands and softens, to allow the descent of the diaphragm.
- The pelvic floor releases and lengthens.

What happens when you breathe out?

- The exhalation expels air from the body.
- The pelvic floor contracts and lifts
- The belly naturally moves inward
- The ribs soften and close, like bellows or an accordion closing, as the lungs empty.

Think: inhale to expand and exhale to engage

Pelvic floor physiotherapy can make a difference with symptoms of incontinence within three months. They can also be helpful for managing and alleviating the symptoms of prolapse. Specifically, six months of supervised pelvic floor muscle training has benefits in terms of anatomical and symptom improvement.[2]

How often should I be doing my pelvic floor exercises?

For treatment of incontinence, the gold standard for pelvic floor exercises is:

- *3 sets of 10-second holds, plus*
- *10 fast contractions at a rate of around one per second*
- *3 times a day*

We need to practise both fast-twitch, with the quick contractions, and slow-twitch activation with the longer holds (see page 18). A 10-second hold seems to allow for muscle fatigue that stimulates the muscles to become stronger. We need to train both sub-maximally and with maximum effort. A max contraction can sometimes elicit a better relaxation response. Make sure when you're reaching your "max" engagement that you're not also clenching other muscles. Think "soft buttocks, soft shoulders, soft eyebrows, soft jaw".

SOME PELVIC FLOOR IMAGERY

- On the inhale, invite your ribs to expand laterally, the belly to inflate softly and the vulva to blossom.
- Imagine your labia like lungs that are filling up with air as you breathe in. Exhale and imagine sipping a smoothie with a straw with your vagina.
- Feel the blossom close and lift. Feel the belly gently engage and draw in as the ribs return to resting.
- Inhale and expand. Now exhale and imagine picking up a blueberry with your vagina and anus.
- Inhale and put the berries back down.
- Exhale and imagine your pelvic floor like a jellyfish propelling to the surface of the ocean.
- Inhale and allow the jellyfish to open and softly float.

> *Find the cue that works best for you and then practise your pelvic floor exercises daily.*

Remembering to "do your pelvic floors"

Making time to do pelvic floor exercises three times a day can be challenging, especially for busy people. But – three 10-second holds, and ten fast contractions is around one minute. Everyone has one minute, three times a day. We *do* find two minutes morning and evening to brush our teeth every day, so finding that essential self-care time *can be done*. Tagging it onto an activity you already do, such as brushing your teeth, waiting for the kettle to boil or waiting for the bus, can be a good way of building it into a habit if it really feels difficult to "find the time".

Building pelvic floor work into functional movement

Learning how to incorporate pelvic floor exercise into daily movement means you can add them to a workout and you can bring them into your activities of daily living like lifting laundry, groceries or small children. Plus … this removes the boredom aspect – which is another big reason why people don't do pelvic floor exercise. Researchers also suggests the possibility of benefit in adding abdominal work to pelvic floor exercise, such as Pilates or Pfilates (see page 147), can increase effectiveness.[3]

HOW DO I INCORPORATE IT INTO MY DAILY MOVEMENT?

"Blow as you go"

When you are doing something which requires a pelvic floor activation, practice consciously engaging into your pelvic floor.

1   When you lift a heavy weight: such as picking your baby up out of the bath, or lifting a carseat/heavy toddler/basket of washing – lift on the exhale, engaging your pelvic floor as you do so.

2   When you are getting up from sitting down or being on the floor, breathe out and lift up into your pelvic floor to assist the movement.

3   When you're about to sneeze or cough, actively lift up into your pelvic floor before you do so, if you have time!

Pelvic floor hypertonicity

Some people may have been told that they have a hypertonic pelvic floor or overactive pelvic floor muscles and should not do "kegels". If this is you, perhaps the *way* you do them, or the focus of your effort needs to be different, but you will still benefit from taking your pelvic floor through the full expression of movement. Some may even benefit by trying to contract their muscle as hard as possible to trigger a subsequent full release.

BLOSSOM BREATHING

Blossom breathing is a good visual for people to imagine a flower opening up. Focus on the inhale, release tension in the whole pelvic floor:

One contract and lift (exhale to engage) for every 3–5 blossom breaths (inhale to expand).

Open up the ribs, soften the belly and release tension in the vulva.

Pelvic floor exercises, contract and release, are a core exercise and are something that we can benefit from *for life*.

Kegel weights

Vaginal weight lifting and the use of yoni eggs has become popular in the last few years, most likely due to the increased awareness about pelvic health through social media. While it is great that more people are searching for options, kegel weights are not the best idea for a first timer and while they can play a valuable role in pelvic floor fitness, they are not for everyone. It is also important that a person has an understanding about the type of training their pelvic floor would benefit from as well as a respect for certain guidelines for kegel weight training. A study comparing pelvic floor exercise with electrical stimulation and vaginal weights (cones) found that improvement is muscle strength was significantly higher after pelvic floor exercises than after electrical stimulation or using vaginal cones.[4]

That's not to say that there is no benefit. My recommendation is to see a pelvic floor physiotherapist first. Before investing in a set of weights or a strengthening device, invest time (or money) in a pelvic floor physiotherapist assessment. Your physiotherapist can help you determine if a device would be beneficial for you and if so, which one may be best and how to use it effectively.

Many people associate things like incontinence, prolapse and unsatisfying sex with weakness and laxity or low tone, but sometimes weakness is a result of overactive muscles or non-relaxing pelvic floor muscles. If this is the case and you choose to buy a set of kegel weights and use them how they are commonly recommended, which is to put them in and walk around or wear them for a workout, your problem may get worse. This can actually lead to more overuse, gripping and overactivity. It can also be discouraging for some who find they can't hold the weight in.

I believe kegel weights have a place, and prefer a timed training session of about ten minutes every day or every other day. I also prefer silicone devices as opposed to stone or crystal eggs. I have heard too many stories from users and from pelvic floor physiotherapists about infection from using the stone and crystal yoni eggs that I believe silicone devices are better suited for repeated use. Intimate Rose is a company founded by pelvic floor physical therapist Dr Amanda Olson and offers a great variety of options and education.

Kegel weights can provide resistance and feedback, which can be helpful for some people. Some therapists use kegel weights with their clients to help them build strength by gently tugging on the inserted weight while asking the patient to resist the pull using their pelvic floor muscles. There are many different shapes and sizes of weights. I don't believe in super heavy weights and do like the ones that offer an element of movement such as the kegelbell and kegel balls or ben-wa-balls. Be sure to use a product that has a cord or tail for easy removal. Many eggs and some devices do not have an option for removal and recommend getting into a squat and bearing down. I do not support this advice and prefer to have people use products with an attached string or tail to avoid bearing down.

A study looking at whole-body vibration training found that whole-body vibration training, with the vSculpt pelvic floor trainer, has beneficial effects in improving pelvic floor muscle strength and quality of life in patients with incontinence.[5]

Pessaries

Pessaries are removeable prosthetic devices inserted into the vagina to help restore pelvic anatomy in the case of organ prolapse and/or aid in reducing or eliminating stress urinary incontinence symptoms. The origin of pessaries dates back to ancient Egypt where they would use earth and honey to treat a "fallen womb". During the time of Hippocrates the uterus was thought to act like an animal unto itself so fumigation treatments would be used in an attempt to get the uterus to retreat. Vinegar-soaked sponges and halved pomegranates were also used. If none of these treatments worked, women were hanged upside down by their feet in an attempt to reposition the falling organ. Next came balls of wool wrapped in linen and soaked in vinegar, then wax and metal, then plastic. Today we have thankfully evolved and there are many different pessary options available and most are made of medical-grade silicone.

Pessaries can be life changing. They can eliminate symptoms and fear associated with prolapse, which gives many people their life back. Some people choose to wear them only during exercise or work, while others wear them daily no matter what. Some pessaries are put in and taken out each day, while others can stay in up to three months. Some pessaries can even be worn during penetrative intercourse. There are some pessaries that can be inserted by the individual themselves and others need to be inserted and removed by a healthcare provider.

Typically pessaries are fitted by a gynaecologist, GP, practice nurse, or specialist nurse or physiotherapist. The Ring pessary is the one most often given as a first try, depending on the type of prolapse. While there are some pessaries that are typically prescribed for certain types of prolapse, it is important to know that we are all different and what works for one person will not always work for another. It can take several attempts to find the right pessary and the right size but when the perfect pessary is found, it can make all the difference. There is a company looking to offer a 3D printed pessary that would be custom made based on each person's anatomy – a fascinating idea which could remove the sometimes lengthy process of finding the right fit.

Fitness and lifestyle

Lifestyle habits and exercise can be contributors to pelvic floor challenges, but they can also be the key to managing them as well. The term "core" started springing up quite regularly in the fitness industry in the early 1990s and has remained a buzzword ever since. What is now shifting is the realization that the core is *so much more* than the abs and the lower back. The pelvic floor is the foundation of the core, and understanding how to properly recruit your pelvic floor to support your movement has been an integral part of movement programmes such as Pilates for the past 30 years. Now there is increasing awareness in other areas of the fitness industry.

The fitness industry has also seen a rise in more intense activity and more and more women and people with a vulva and a vagina have been pursuing these activities. CrossFit put out a video in 2013 titled *"CrossFit – Do You Pee During Workouts?"* It highlighted the fact that many female CrossFit athletes leak urine during their WODs (workouts of the day). They used a term EIUL – exercise-induced urinary leakage. It is also sometimes called light bladder leakage but the truth is, it is incontinence. The video suggests that leaking is "just what it takes to be the fittest woman on the planet".

There was even a gynaecologist who said, "We need to invent something to help these women" and then went on to say that in her professional opinion "It is ok to pee during double unders" (double unders are a common exercise in CrossFit where you skip with a rope and do two rotations of the rope instead of one during the skip). I am NOT OK with her statement. **Leaking urine is NOT normal. It is a very clear indication that something is not working as it should be and the signals will only get louder until you stop and listen to your body and do something about it.**

CrossFit has been an incredible community for many. Their website states that the CrossFit essentials are, "constantly varied high-intensity functional movement coupled with meat and vegetables, nuts and seeds, some fruit, little starch and no sugar – prepares you for the demands of a healthy, functional, independent life and provides a hedge against chronic disease and incapacity." I love this and love the variety of movements, the community and the sense of accomplishment that people feel. What I struggle with is the intensity of some of the workouts, and the CrossFit culture of pushing your body beyond comfortable limits. The community aspect is motivating, but it can also create a sense of pressure to perform and sometimes people may push the boundaries a bit too much. This goes for any activity, not just CrossFit.

I appreciate that CrossFit is inclusive, however bodies with a vulva and a vagina are different than those without, especially if those bodies have given birth. Pregnancy and birth heighten the differences and the need for alternatives that are not always supported in the WOD.

Fitness should feed your mind and body and fuel your confidence and self-esteem. Activities that bring about sensations of heaviness or leaking are in essence robbing you of some of that. Women leaking urine during exercise are also leaking power and potential. When the pelvic floor and inner core system are working synergistically, the leaks stop and the power increases.

CASE STUDY – SHELLY (30)

I met Shelly when she was eight months postpartum with her first child. She had been an avid runner before giving birth and had dealt with IBS since she was a teen. After the birth of her baby she was having challenges controlling her IBS and was often not able to make it to the bathroom in time. She had returned to running but was too afraid to run outdoors in case there was no bathroom, so she was running at home on the treadmill wearing incontinence briefs.

We worked together over four sessions. We reviewed posture and breathing. Her homework from the first session was to practise the core breath and check in with her posture a few times a day. She had a lot of tension in her posterior pelvic floor and had been working with a pelvic health physio but had reached a plateau.

At the second session, she was feeling more confident about her posture and her core breath so we added it to some movements. She left with the bridge, squats, bicep curls and one-leg stand for exercises to practise with her core breath.

In the third session, I taught her three hypopressive poses, which was her homework in addition to progressions of the last exercises.

During her fourth session, she said she was feeling some changes and was starting to notice more control. I taught her the rest of the hypopressive poses and gave her some more advanced progressions for strength training for running.

She messaged me a couple of months later to let me know that she was running outside without the incontinence briefs! She was elated and even said she was running faster and longer than she was before baby! I was so happy for her and proud of her for putting in the work – her commitment and consistency paid off big time!

A few years ago I was teaching my Core Confidence Specialist Certification course at a large fitness conference and there was a physiotherapist in the group who was asking a lot of questions and doubting a lot of what my partners and I were teaching. The day after the course she came up to us after one of our presentations and said "Okay, I'm convinced. I used the core breath in my workout this morning and the nagging knee pain I had in my lunge was gone and I was also able to lift more weight in my shoulder press." She was elated as she understood how powerful the breath and pelvic floor synergy can be.

The pelvis is our powerhouse and when we can harness its full potential we can soar to new heights! This is true if you are currently struggling with incontinence or prolapse, or have no symptoms at all.

Antony Lo is a physiotherapist in Australia who has been a huge catalyst for change with regards to fitness for people with pelvic floor dysfunction. He questions everything and challenges the beliefs that are so often holding people back from living their best life. He has been instrumental in shifting the perspectives about lifting and movement for people living with core challenges like prolapse and diastasis recti.

When these conditions were first talked about on social media, there were many do's and don'ts lists. Safe and unsafe exercises limited people and I believe contributed to the depressive symptoms many people felt. Rather than state that an exercise is bad or take something away from a person, Antony seeks to see how the person can "do it differently". This has fuelled a whole new perspective for pelvic health professionals and trainers and is helping shift the pendulum to allow for a variety of options with an individualized approach.

Moving in varied ways is hugely beneficial, but sometimes we get stuck in fitness ruts where we only do one or two things. Then when a pelvic floor issue appears and threatens to put an end to those one or two activities it can feel like the end of the world. I invite you to be curious and see how you can "do it differently". Can you do it slower? Fewer repetitions? Can you alter the pace? Lighten the load? Can you do it less often? Change the range of motion? Can you use a different core cue? Change the time of day you do it? Can you alter your breath pattern? There really are so many options to modify a movement or activity and if after trying them, your symptoms do not improve or reduce then perhaps there is another exercise that will serve you better. Always ask yourself *why* you are doing an exercise. What is your goal? Then self-assess and decide if the movement or exercise is taking you toward your goal or not. It may not be, but you may love the exercise and not want to give it up. That is your choice and if it is an informed one then go for it!

I promote high-intensity interval training (HIIT) but not every day, especially not for early postpartum parents and people in menopause. Repetitive high-intensity workouts can be a stressor, can raise cortisol levels and can deplete the adrenals that are already near their end range. Do two to three HIIT workouts coupled with walks, yoga and weight-bearing exercise each week. Something I also recommend three to four times a week is hypopressives.

Hypopressives

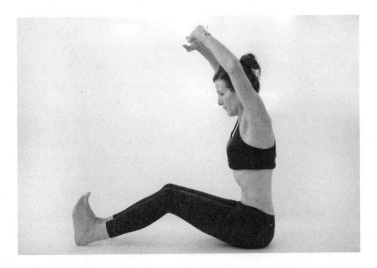

I first learned about hypopressives from Kasia Tuominen. She was promoting an unfamiliar-looking technique that was supposed to help with incontinence and prolapse. I was intrigued and began following her work, tried to replicate what she was doing, and subsequently trained to teach the technique. I became committed to practising regularly after I was told my uterus was moving south! I reversed a uterine prolapse within a few months and have been practising four to five times a week ever since.

The term "hypopressive" means "low pressure" and the technique is now often called "low pressure fitness". For those who are familiar with Uddiyana Bandha from yoga or the abdominal vacuum from bodybuilding, hypopressives is similar and has been expanded into a full fitness programme that has potential – which is as yet not backed up with clinical evidence – for postural re-education, abdominal wall tone and function, incontinence, organ prolapse and even pelvic pain. Those who have more laxity may notice an increase in tone while those who are hypertonic or have overactive muscles may notice a decrease in tone.

The technique involves a series of postures which are considered low pressure, meaning they do not create an increase in intra-abdominal pressure. A rhythmic breathing pattern is added including a period of breath-holding called an "apnea". The apnea is done at the end of a full exhalation and is also called a "false breath". Essentially you exhale all of your air, close your glottis (some need to use a nose plug or physically plug their own nose when first learning) and then hold the breath. The intercostal muscles expand the ribs, which mimics what the ribs do on an inhalation. Because there is no air coming it creates a negative pressure response which draws the relaxed diaphragm up and the abdomen is passively drawn in. The suction effect influences the intra-thoracic, intra-abdominal and intro-pulmonic pressures. It draws the pelvic viscera up and leads to a myofascial release of the pelvic floor structures.

See more about Hypopressives in the Appendix, page 149.

CASE STUDY – KELLY (30)

Kelly sought my help when she was nine months post-birth and had been diagnosed with a grade 3 bladder prolapse

---

(also called a cystocele). She had read about hypopressives in a prolapse forum and was searching for someone to help her learn the technique to see if she could improve her prolapse and reduce or eliminate her symptoms.

Kelly gave birth vaginally after a fast labour (five hours total) and 1.5 hours of pushing. She birthed her baby in a hospital in the lithotomy position (lying on her back) holding her legs. She had an epidural but was not assisted with vacuum or forceps. She experienced a second-degree tear.

She saw a pelvic floor physio at six weeks postpartum and also had an IUD inserted by her doctor around the same time. Kelly is very active with running, climbing and weight-lifting so returned to her regular fitness routine.

At four months she felt "a dropping sensation" during exercise and knew immediately that she had a prolapse. Kelly works in the medical field and already knew about prolapse but never thought it would happen to her.

During our first online session I evaluated her posture and did some movement assessments with her. She had a common post-pregnancy posture that has a forward presentation of the pelvis with a posterior tilt. She was also very rounded in the shoulders and her upper back was leaning backward. This meant her weight was very much in her forefeet, her diaphragm and pelvic floor were not in their optimal alignment and her glute muscles were inhibited. I gave her some verbal cues to help her find a more neutral posture and she noticed immediately that her prolapse symptoms (heaviness and pressure) improved. This was a huge eye opener for her and allowed her to become very conscious of how she held her body, especially while holding her child.

I guided her through a self-assessment of her abdomen and she did not have a significant gap and felt tension in the connective tissue when she performed a pelvic floor contraction.

Her main goal was to learn hypopressives, so I taught her the basics of the apnea (the breath-hold part of the hypopressive posture), which she connected with right away. I then fine-tuned the posture with the appropriate arm and leg positions, as well as added cues for elongating the spine and expanding the ribs. I gave her three poses to practise every other day until our next session.

I followed up with her after a week and she had done a self-check and noticed that her prolapse was higher than usual – she was elated and very motivated!

During her first follow up which was three weeks later she said she was "net neutral". She had developed a really bad cough but had been diligent with the hypopressives and there was no worsening of her symptoms. Overall she loved the feeling of doing hypopressives and found that the day following her hypopressive exercises she felt better. She had little to no heaviness and definitely noticed fewer symptoms. I gave her an additional three poses.

During her second follow up, two weeks later, her cough was gone and she was doing the six poses every other day along with voluntary pelvic floor exercises (kegels). She had good and bad days, but overall felt an improvement and was noticing that the "feeling like there is a tampon in there" sensation was happening less and less. She was also fitted for a cube pessary at this time. She had tried a few ring pessaries with no success and was hopeful the cube would be better.

I checked in with her a week after our second session and she had tried the cube and felt it helped a bit but did notice some cramping. She kept up with her hypopressives (she was doing four to five days a week now) and was noticing big improvements. Even on days when she was babywearing and hiking, she noticed few, if any, symptoms later in the day – a huge win.

In the third session I gave her some lifting-technique advice, some fine tuning on some of the kegel exercises she was doing as well as a few additional hypopressive poses.

At her fourth and final session she had been to see her pelvic floor physio who reported an improvement in her kegels (more lift) and the prolapse had reduced by at least a stage. Kelly also did an apnea while the physio assessed her pelvic floor and could hardly believe how much of a lift she got.

Kelly was elated and was so empowered! She had a new exercise regime that she loved but that also helped. She no longer felt like her exercise life was over and she had greatly reduced her symptoms.

Surgery

Surgery can be life changing and is absolutely needed *in some cases*. It is often offered as the "only solution" and sometimes before the conservative treatment options have been explored fully. Knowledge about pelvic floor function and the need for pre-hab and re-hab can improve surgical outcomes and potentially prevent the possibility of recurrence while improving the longevity of the surgery.

There are many different surgeries available and there are some key points to keep in mind while making a decision to have surgery that could ensure satisfaction.

When being referred to a surgeon, it is often based on your nearest hospital. Asking your pelvic floor physiotherapist who they recommend is always a good idea. They see the work of the surgeons, the good and the bad outcomes, so can help direct you to who they would recommend. You can do online searches and look at doctor ratings to help you make your choice so you can narrow your options down. When you see your family doctor you can then ask for a referral to your first choice. Keep in mind that you can choose to ask for another referral if you are not happy with your first choice. On the day of your appointment with the surgeon, be prepared with your questions and if you don't feel comfortable with the person, ask for a referral to the next person on your list. Do this until you feel comfortable with the person who will be doing the surgery. Being informed gives your control and confidence.

Here are some questions to ask your surgeons:

- Do I need surgery?
- What is the name of the surgical procedure you are recommending?
- Do I need surgery now?
- Is there harm in waiting?
- What are the alternatives to surgery?
- Are there other surgeries, maybe less invasive?
- Why this one over the alternatives?
- Will you use mesh or native tissue?
- Is it done laparascopically or as open surgery?
- What kind of anesthesia will be used?
- How long will the procedure take?
- What is the success rate? What is YOUR success rate?
- What are some of the possible negative outcomes?
- What complications are there?
- What are the risks?
- What results can I expect?
- How long will the results last?
- How long is the recovery? How long will I stay in hospital?
- What do I need to do to prepare?
- When can I return to work?
- When can I return to exercise?

Bring your list and write down the answers. If you're within a private healthcare framework, you may want to interview another to get a second opinion (this would not be an option within the NHS). Being as informed as you possibly can is of utmost importance.

Once you have made your decision and scheduled your surgery it is important to optimize your bowel movements, work with a pelvic floor physio, support your immune system and get lots of rest in preparation. Stay active and keep up with your pelvic floor muscle training.

It is important to keep in mind that surgery will restore the anatomy for the most part but if the things that led to the development of the problem in the first place are not addressed, the chance of recurrence is high. Optimizing bowel habits and elimination is key, ensuring the pelvic floor muscles are working in a balanced way (contract and relax), synergizing the breath with the pelvic floor, learning to manage intra-abdominal pressure and working with a pelvic floor physiotherapist and personal trainer to fine-tune your movement are all good ideas if you can. Many times, people have surgery and are freed by the elimination of symptoms so they return or start high-intensity exercise once they are cleared by their clincian. If, however, they have not learned to activate their pelvic floor and coordinate with their breath and bring it into movement, they could end up needing another surgical procedure.

CASE STUDY – SARAH (58)

Sarah was a participant in one of my 28-day challenges and had great results, so she asked me to work with her one-on-one to help her progress.

She was struggling with some SI joint pain and some feelings of heaviness from a uterine prolapse. She was advised by one surgeon to "just take it out" but she really did not need more surgery. She had had a cystocele and rectocele repair in 2010 and did not want to have to go through that again.

Sarah had had four vaginal births and an episiotomy with three of them. She did not experience any pelvic pain or incontinence. It was mainly SI joint pain on occasion and feelings of heaviness from the prolapse.

She had worked with another trainer and had learned hypopressives and was doing them three times a week, as well as the exercises she had learned in my challenge. She also did yoga, walked, swam and cycled (I do love active people!).

During our first session I began with posture and movement assessments. Her posture was pretty good – just a few small adjustments and cues to help her release some tension in her bum and posterior pelvic floor. I fine-tuned a couple of things with her hypopressives and gave her a couple of alternative poses to try. I also noticed she had a breath holding and bearing-down strategy when doing some of the exercises, so I worked with her to change that and then had her practise the pelvic tilt, squats, bird dog and bicep curls. She had been avoiding weights because she was afraid of making her prolapse worse.

At her first follow up she said she felt great! Had no SI joint pain and felt no heaviness with any of the exercises. I counselled her on her pessary and suggested she use it more often as it reduces symptoms but may also help improve the recruitment of muscles when she exercises.

In her second follow up we added a few more weighted exercises, paying close attention to form and her breathing. She had a tendency to go quite fast, so we found a 2-up/2-down count for her that seemed to help her maintain a consistent rate and not use momentum.

During her third session she reported that she was doing her weight training every other day and was feeling stronger with no symptoms, even when she wasn't wearing the pessary.

During her fourth session she remarked that she had experienced a bit of sacrum pain, so I modified a few exercises and gave her a few new release exercises. I suggested she do the piriformis release and posterior pelvic floor release before and after each workout.

I continue to work with her on a bi-weekly basis as she likes the accountability. She is now doing jump squats, dynamic rear lunges with kicks, ball push-ups and combo moves such as squats with bicep curls. She is making huge progress and was also excited as she had a new man in her life and her confidence was greatly improved because of the work she had put in.

Clothing

I am fortunate to work in fitness so my wardrobe is activewear pretty much every day. I have worked in corporate jobs where I wore a suit and heels every day and I will never go back. When I put on clothing other than activewear I realize how much what I wear dictates how I move. From footwear to undies to bras and tank tops, what we wear may have an effect on our posture, breath – and possibly pelvic health.

I was a runner for close to 15 years before experiencing nagging knee pain (classic IT band syndrome) right before I became pregnant with my first child. I didn't run during my pregnancy and when I tried to return after my baby was born the pain was still there. I then began a journey of various health treatments to try and "fix" my knee. Nothing seemed to work until I transitioned to barefoot shoes. I bought my first pair of Vibram 5 fingers close to 13 years ago and they made a huge difference in my feet, my knees and my back when standing all day at a tradeshow. Standing all day in Vibram's – there was no back pain. Standing all day in classic running shoes – major back pain. Recently I have added another brand Altra to the mix and love the freedom my feet have to move. Regular shoes "cast" our feet, a term I learned from Katy Bowman (author of *Move Your DNA*, among other wonderful books). The narrow toe boxes of most footwear restricts the movement of the toes and the intrinsic musculature in the feet. This translates up the chain and can influence our knees, hips, back and pelvic floor.

When you get dressed tomorrow and throughout the day, ask yourself how each piece of clothing you choose affects your body. Maybe you have a tight pair of trousers or jeans on, or perhaps a pencil skirt. Can you take long walking strides? Can you squat down to pick something up? I'll answer that for you now. Nope. What you wear can either facilitate or restrict your movement, and tight clothing can exacerbate that even more, especially shapewear. Clothing that is tight or compressive in the waist can hinder breath and digestion, and can possibly create downward pressure on the pelvic floor. See how you can liberate your body with different choices. Clothing that allows you to stretch, to sit in neutral, to squat, to bend, to rotate. We need variability in our movement, and wearing clothing that moves with you will change your life.

CHAPTER 7
MOVEMENT AND EXERCISE

Movement is absolutely crucial for optimizing pelvic floor function. But it can be the one thing that is actively avoided because people are afraid to leak or they are afraid of making their problem worse.

Exercise is important, as is regular habitual movement. *They are different.* Someone who sits at a desk all day and then goes to the gym for an hour may have enough "exercise", but across the board doesn't have a lot of movement. A term used by one of my teachers Katy Bowman is "nutritious movement". We need a *variety of movement* in the same way that we need a variety of foods, so one thing you can start with is to look at your day.

- How much movement do you get?
- How could you get more?
- How could you vary it?
- Could you add regular, short "movement snacks" into a day that was otherwise quite sedentary?

It could be as simple as sitting on the floor for part of your work day, standing for part of it, walking for part of it and sitting in a chair for part of it. It could mean doing some stretches at your desk every hour. It could be taking a walking conference call.

Make sure that you don't find yourself sitting still for longer than an hour at a time.

Move more. Sit less.

We shouldn't look at exercise as a way to make up for the lack of movement we have in our day, or as a punishment. Exercise and movement are gifts and they are essential nutrients for our body. They are also a huge part of overcoming pelvic floor dysfunction.

As people with female anatomy and hormones, we need to mind our intensity as it pertains to cortisol production, hormone balance and pelvic floor symptoms. We benefit from bone loading and short HIIT workouts two to three times per week, as well as yoga and meditation to help with stress management.

I invite you to let go of the pressure to train hard, or flip tires or do 20 box jumps. If you want to do those things, and your body is able to manage the loads, then you absolutely can but I don't believe they are serving us fully. The intensity can often deplete rather than build us – and when you add pelvic floor dysfunction into the mix the depletion can seem more significant.

Learn your ABCs

My general rule of thumb is to focus on the ABCs. Optimize your ALIGNMENT, connect with your BREATH, and perform CONSISTENT and COORDINATED movement. Releasing non-optimal patterns can help improve alignment, so I always start with down training/release exercises. This often facilitates the connection to the breath. Once the breath (core breath) is more fluid and you have a sense of connection with your breath and pelvic floor, then you add in movements that incorporate the pelvic floor and are heightened by adding in the core breath. It is a bit of retraining that then progresses to training.

Retrain before you train

Retraining is generally defined as the renewal or updating of skills. It is always my first step for anyone who has recently given birth, anyone currently dealing with incontinence, prolapse, back pain and/or diastasis recti. We need to connect before we can correct. Unfortunately, by exercising blindly without an understanding of our inner core, and by loading the core or the body when that inner core is not working properly, we miss out on power potential, on load transfer and core control.

One of my favourite sayings from Paul Chek is, "You can't fire a cannon from a canoe," which so clearly illustrates the new mums at bootcamp classes who have waited for the six-week green light and have then gone from 0–60 too quickly. It illustrates the many people in high-intensity fitness classes who could better achieve their goals by turning inward first.

What needs to happen first, ideally, is a reconnection of sorts. We need to remind the body about the relationship between the diaphragm and the pelvic floor, and then slowly add it to movement that helps us build back up to what we used to do. *We need to retrain before we train.* Retraining helps reestablish the connection to the pelvic floor that is often lost due to stretched abdominal muscles, nerve interruption in the pelvic floor, poor posture, childbirth, accidents, surgeries, falls and even trauma.

Retraining involves resetting the foundation for proper Alignment, Breathing and Coordination (ABC). And then progressing to training which is recognized as an important factor in improved performance. Once we have retrained, we then use progressive loads to train the core.

Pelvic floor retraining exercises

Down-training exercises

Down training is essentially learning to let go of stuck tension and restriction that may be hindering optimal pelvic floor function and posture. These are "allowing" exercises ... not "doing" exercises.

Posterior pelvic floor release

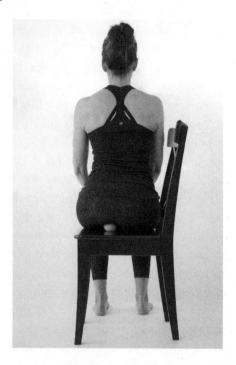

- Have a tennis ball in hand and then sit in a neutral pelvis position on a hard-surfaced chair.
- Lift up your right bum cheek and place the ball in the area between your anus and your sit bone.
- Lower the buttock back down.
- Imagine the ball is a strawberry and your buttock muscles are melting chocolate.
- Your goal is to cover the strawberry with chocolate.
- Hold for 30 seconds.
- Repeat on other side.
- Do 1–2 times/day.

Supine butterfly

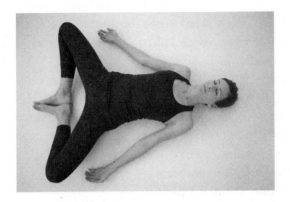

- Lie on your back on the floor with your knees bent.
- Allow your knees to gently fall out to the sides and place the soles of your feet together.
- If you have a lot of tightness in your hips and inner thighs you may benefit from putting some towels or pillows underneath your thighs so you can release into the pose.
- Stay here for 1–2 minutes.

Standing hamstring release

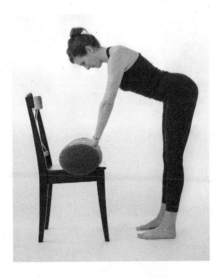

- Place a stack of towels or some blocks on a chair.
- Stand in front of the chair with your feet hip-width apart and your pelvis parallel with the ground.
- Hinge at your hips and place your straight arms on top of the stack of blocks or towels.
- Ensure you keep a gentle curve in your lower back and imagine your sit bones floating up to the sky.
- If you don't feel much release or stretch, take out one of the blocks but ensure you don't tuck in your tailbone.
- Keep your neck neutral or let your head hang.
- Hold for 30–60 seconds.
- Do multiple times a day.

Thoracic release

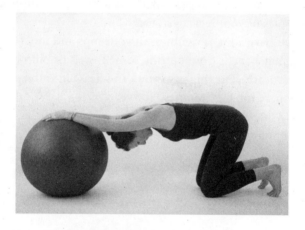

- Kneel on the floor in front of a stability ball, couch or ottoman.
- Place your hands and forearms on the surface of your ball or furniture.
- You can stay kneeling with your bottom on your heels or you can lift your bottom off your heels.
- Imagine your sit bones floating up to the sky.
- Keep your lower ribs in line with the top of your pelvis and prevent them from thrusting forward.

- Hold for 30–60 seconds.
- Do multiple times a day.

Beginner up training

Up training is about building strength, endurance and coordination. Once you learn and practise the core breath you will progress by adding the core breath to movements that will really fire up your core and activate your power centre.

Core breath

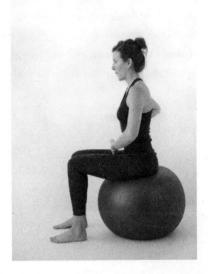

- Sit on a stability ball or straddle a bolster.
- Find neutral pelvis with your vulva on the surface of the bolster or ball and your tailbone lengthening out from under you. You should feel a gentle curve in the lower back.
- Place one hand on your side ribs and one hand on your belly.

- Inhale and send your breath laterally into your ribs and feel a small overflow in the belly. Allow your ribs and belly to expand.
- Direct your attention to your pelvic floor on the ball or bolster. As you inhale, feel a sense of fullness on the surface of the ball or bolster. Imagine your vulva blossoming.
- Now exhale and imagine picking up a blueberry with your vagina and anus. You can also try other imagery such as sipping a smoothie through a straw with your vagina, preventing a tampon from slipping out, imagine a string |on your perineum and gently pull it up to the crown of your head.
- Inhale and expand again.
- Repeat for 30–60 seconds.
- Remember, **inhale to expand, exhale to engage**. After you practise and perfect the core breath you will then add it to these movements.

Core breath with pelvic tilt

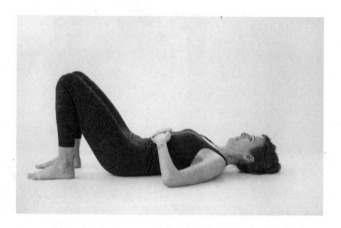

- Lie on your back with your knees bent.
- Have a small towel under your head if needed to keep your neck in neutral.

- Ensure you have a neutral pelvis by placing the heel of your hands on your hip bones and your fingertips on your pubic joint. They should be in an even plane. If your fingertips are higher, you are in a posterior tilt and need to increase the arch in the low back slightly while nodding the pubic joint toward the floor. If the heels of your hands are higher, you are in an exaggerated anterior tilt and need to allow the low back to move toward the floor (do not flatten completely) and your pubic joint to float back toward your belly button slightly.
- Now add the core breath to the movement.
- **Inhale to expand, exhale to engage** and then press the low back into the floor as your pelvis tilts backward.
- Inhale to expand as you return to neutral pelvis.
- Repeat 10 times.

Core breath with bridge

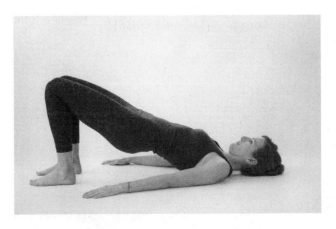

- Lie on your back with your knees bent and your shins vertical.
- Have a small towel under your head if needed to keep your neck in neutral.
- Ensure you have a neutral pelvis by placing the heel of your hands on your hip bones and your fingertips on your pubic

joint. They should be in an even plane. If your fingertips are higher, you are in a posterior tilt and need to increase the arch in the low back slightly while nodding the pubic joint toward the floor. If the heels of your hands are higher, you are in an exaggerated anterior tilt and need to allow the low back to move toward the floor (do not flatten completely) and your pubic joint to float back toward your belly button slightly.

- Now add the core breath to the movement.
- **Inhale to expand, exhale to engage** and then lift your bum off the floor.
- Inhale to expand as you lower back down to start.
- Ideally you do not tilt the pelvis in this movement, however at the start you may find it easier to do so.
- Repeat 10 times.

Intermediate up training

Core breath with bent knee side plank

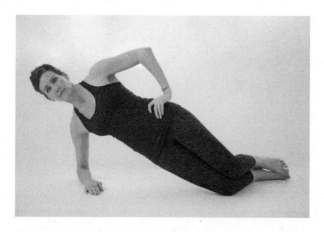

- Sit on your side with your knees bent at a 45-degree angle and your heels in line with your bum.
- Check in to make sure you have a gentle curve in your lower back.

- Lower your upper body to the mat so you are resting on a bent arm with your elbow under your shoulder
- **Inhale to expand then exhale to engage**, then press your pelvis forward while lifting your hip off the
- Inhale to expand as you lower back down.
- Repeat 10 times per side.

Core breath with seated march

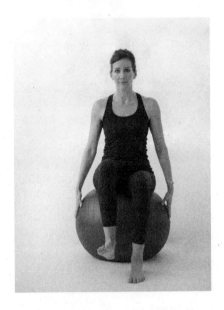

- Sit on a stability ball or hard-surfaced chair.
- Find neutral pelvis with your vulva on the surface of the bolster or ball and your tailbone out from under you. You should feel a gentle curve in the lower back.
- Place your hands at your sides – you may wish to place your hands on the side of the ball if you are using one.
- **Inhale to expand, exhale to engage**, then lift your right foot off the ground about 1–2 inches.
- Inhale to expand as you return the foot to the ground.
- Repeat 10 times per side.

Core breath with one-leg stand

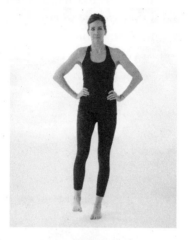

- Stand with feet pelvis width apart.
- **Inhale to expand then exhale to engage** and slowly transfer your weight to your right foot while lifting the left foot off the ground 1–2 inches.
- Inhale to expand as you put the foot back down.
- Repeat 10 times on each side.

Advanced up training

Core breath with squat

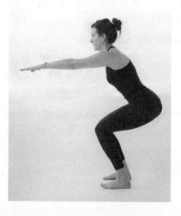

- Stand with feet pelvis width apart.
- Inhale to expand as your lower yourself down into a squat. Initiate the movement by hinging at your hips and sending your bum backwards.
- At the lowest point of your squat (you choose your desired range of motion) exhale to engage and stand back up.
- Repeat 10 times.

Core breath with lunge

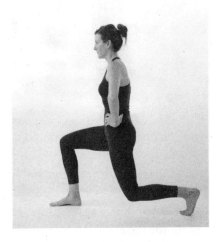

- Stand in a staggered stance with your left leg behind you, heel lifted and toes firmly planted.
- Your right leg will be slightly bent.
- Inhale to expand as you lower your body down into a lunge.
- At the lowest point of your lunge (you choose your desired range of motion) exhale to engage and stand back up.
- Ensure you are moving up and down in the centre as opposed to allowing your weight to shift forward over your front knee.
- Repeat 10 times.

Core breath with deadlift

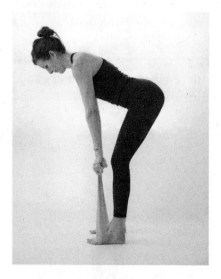

- Stand with your feet pelvis width apart and a small bend in the knees.
- Place a theraband underneath your feet and hang on to each end with your hands.
- Inhale to expand as you hinge at your hips and allow your upper body to tip forward.
- Exhale to engage as you return to start ensuring your keep a long torso and do not round in your back.
- Repeat 10 times.

CHAPTER 8
FREQUENTLY ASKED QUESTIONS AND FINAL TIPS

We have covered a lot and perhaps you are feeling a litte overwhelmed. Or, hopefully you have found some clarity and now have some tools you can use in your life to take control of your pelvic health. Below is a list of the most common questions I get. Questions that maybe you still have.

Frequently asked questions

Do I need to do pelvic floor exercises every day?
In a word, yes. Evidence suggests three times a day for maintenance and up to six times a day if you have a challenge to overcome. If you are looking to maintain continence and function, aim for at least *something* once a day.

And remember, you can incorporate your pelvic floor exercises into your activities of daily living and your workouts too.

Should I add pelvic floor awareness to my cardio too?

Pelvic floor exercises are best done on their own in seated, lying or standing position or with weights and slower movements. Once you start speeding up, it's less easy to add pelvic floor exercises. Remember the pelvic floor moves in coordination with the diaphragm. As our breathing increases, that dance between them increases and to try and coordinate inhale to expand and exhale to engage at that speed is a bit of a challenge.

Is it too late for me?

If you are alive then it is not too late. *It is never too late.* We have amazing bodies that are capable of changing and evolving and healing no matter our age or stage or history.

How long will it take for me to see results?

It depends. I know how frustrating this answer is, but it depends on a few things: your history; your current pelvic floor function; your goals.

But really it depends most on your commitment to doing the work needed. Small changes done over time can lead to big results. It only takes about 10 minutes a day (maybe 20 if you are doing hypopressives and pelvic floor exercises). Staying consistent is key and will yield results. I have seen people notice results in as little as a week, but 2–3 weeks is most common. I have also seen what happens when people get results, achieve a goal and then stop doing the work. The symptoms come back. It is a lifestyle, not a quick fix.

Can I do crunches?

I don't know. Can you? What is your goal? Are you seeing results? Do you feel symptoms later in the day or the day following? Could you do them differently? Are there alternatives?

You can ask yourself this question about any exercise. What is your goal, what is your execution of the exercise of choice and what are your symptoms? Then you can decide if the exercise is taking you toward or away from your goal.

Stu McGill is probably one of the most closely associated researchers to crunches, and he has shown that there is a detrimental effect to intradiscal pressure during crunches. He also showed that crunches actually only use 20% of rectus abdominis potential.

From an efficiency perspective, we want to get maximum results, so if there was another exercise that would recruit closer to 100% of rectus, do you think that may be a better option? Again, it's about informed choice. If you love crunches, then do them. My tips for execution would be to keep your pelvis in neutral, exhale to engage your pelvic floor and transversus first, and then add in your crunch. Monitor your symptoms doing the exercise and after ... how do you feel? Do you know the risks? Do the risks outweigh the benefits to them? Do you care? Are you making an informed choice?

Final thoughts and tips

If we want something to change, we need to change something. It is my sincere wish that you take what you have learned from this book and put it into practice and then tell others to do the same. It takes a village and below are some of my final tips as well as pelvic health wisdom from some of my favourite pelvic health peeps around the world.

Do the maths

If you use incontinence pads, determine what you spend on them each month and then multiply that by 12, and then by how many years you have left to live (I know we don't know our exact date but I'm hoping to reach at least 100 which means I have around 51 years left).

I did an estimate based on spending $30/month (£15) on light panty liners for 51 years. It was close to $20,000 (£10,000) spent on pads! Not to mention the horrendous cost to the environment. Also consider, that many use more than one light panty liner per day, which increases the cost significantly.

Think about what you could do with 20K, 30K, even 50K!

Book in to see a pelvic floor physiotherapist
Just do it. Put down the book and go make an appointment. It will change your life.

Walk every day
For your body, mind and pelvic floor spirit.

Build your pelvic health team
I have mentioned a few times the benefits of having a pelvic health team. My top picks are:

Pelvic floor physio – see one for as long as you need to, to manage your symptoms, and consider their programme an ongoing one as maintenance even when you are asymptomatic.
Urogynaecologist – annually (may not be possible on the NHS) or as needed.
Doula – if pregnant.
Personal trainer – look for: Core Confidence Education, Burrell Education, Girls Gone Strong, The Centre for Women's Fitness, MuTu System and Adore Your Floor.
Chinese medicine doctor – for hormone balancing, help with digestion and constipation and possibly acupuncture.
Naturopathic doctor – for hormone testing, thyroid testing, digestion, stress management and more.
Holistic nutritionist – for food sensitivity guidance, meal planning for hormonal health, period management and digestion. Also for determining reactive foods such as high histamine foods or inflammatory foods that may trigger pelvic floor symptoms.
Counsellor or psychologist – for help processing a diagnosis, for assistance with birth or other trauma and for overall mental wellbeing.

LIVE A PELVIC-CENTRIC LIFESTYLE

As the owners of vulvas and vaginas we benefit from daily, holistic pelvic floor wellness.

- Remember the "Knack" (see pages 27–28) which is a pre-contraction of the pelvic floor. You can use the knack prior to a cough or sneeze, before you pick something up, or if you feel a strong urge to pee and aren't near a bathroom.
- Use the Squeezy app, which is a multi-award-winning app that supports people with their pelvic floor muscle exercise programmes.
- Staying hydrated is key. Start each day with a glass of water. Then continue to drink regularly throughout the day. This will keep your bladder happy and your stools soft, which will keep your pelvic floor happy.
- I do recommend a dedicated time for pelvic floor exercise practice each day, but sometimes that can be daunting. Doing a set seated or lying on the floor first thing each morning can set the tone for you being more aware for the rest of the day.
- Add a sticky note to your bathroom mirror or by your coffee maker (do them while your coffee is brewing … but a gentle reminder that caffeine can be irritating to the bladder so pay attention to your symptoms).
- You can incorporate pelvic floor exercises into your daily activities like your workouts, standing up from a chair, picking things up, standing in a queue, etc… which makes them much more functional. When you add pelvic floor exercise to movement (which is typically when pelvic floor symptoms happen), you train your pelvic floor to respond to the task at hand.
- Eat foods that are good for YOUR body. Many foods can contribute to inflammation in the body – even seemingly

healthy foods. Using the bladder diary can help as can working with a holistic nutritionist to eliminate foods that contribute to inflammation and bladder irritation. The most common are gluten, dairy, spicy foods, acidic foods, soy, alcohol, caffeine and sugar. Your hormones will be better balanced, your energy more stable, your poos softer and easier to pass and fewer triggers to have to go pee.

- Masturbation is a form of pelvic floor exercise, and when you do pelvic floor exercises while you are participating in self-pleasure it can heighten the sensation.
- Wear clothing that allows you to move freely. So often we move based on what our clothes allow us to do.
- Sit less. Move more and move in varied ways.
- Stretch your calves and hamstrings daily.

APPENDIX 1: MOVEMENT METHODS TO TRAIN THE PELVIC FLOOR – PFILATES AND HYPROPRESSIVES

Pfilates

There is evidence to suggest that movement-based practices can be hugely beneficial in treating urinary incontinence. At the moment, the evidence points at keep doing consistent pelvic floor rehabilitation alongside other activities such as yoga, Pilates and Pfilates (see below), rather than relying on them as a "cure" in themselves. And, as always – don't be scared or feel it's a taboo. Always go to your healthcare provider and request the best course of action with a pelvic health physio.

One of my teachers is Dr Bruce Crawford, a urogynaecologist from Reno, Nevada. I met him on Twitter and was elated to find someone, especially a medical doctor, who was looking at the pelvic floor as part of a team and using fitness to improve function. Before I found his programme, called Pfilates (short for pelvic floor Pilates), everything I was reading about pelvic floor exercise was focused on isolating the pelvic floor. That didn't make sense to me. While I understand that the pelvic floor must be trained without over-activation of other muscles, I didn't believe it worked in isolation. Dr Crawford's work highlighted the glutes, the transversus abdominis and the inner thighs as well as the pelvic floor that all worked together to manage movement. He measured over 150 different exercises to see which ones activated the pelvic floor the most and at what point in the movement was it most activated – he called this "peak engagement." He also measured the activity of the three other muscle groups I mentioned to illustrate that the pelvic floor is not working in isolation and suggested that perhaps movements that harnessed all of these muscle groups could be more beneficial in managing incontinence and prolapse.

I went to his lab in Reno because I wanted to experience his research methods myself. I had wireless EMGs placed on my inner thighs, my glutes, my abdomen and the space between the vagina and anus (perineum) to measure the activity of these muscles in movement. I was then filmed doing various exercises that I could then watch back on a screen that displayed my video as well as my muscle activity during the exercises. I tried various exercises as he prescribed them and then I experimented by adding in the core breath. This really enhanced muscle activity, which excited me because I had been training myself and my clients with the core breath for a couple of years and it was the foundation of my programmes. To see it make a difference was very cool! Dr Crawford chose the ten exercises that elicited the best recruitment of the pelvic floor and then added voluntary contractions to the point of peak engagement of each of those exercises. He uses slow steady holds as well as quick contract/relax cycles at the point of peak engagement to involve more muscle activity.

I also watched videos from other test participants and the one that fascinated me the most was a woman standing in tree pose. She was stable and steady … until she wasn't. She started to lose her balance and tip over. What was so interesting was that milliseconds before she fell, her pelvic floor activity shot up on the EMG recording. It was a perfect illustration of the anticipatory element of the pelvic floor! It knew she was going to fall before she actually did and it fired in anticipation of her needing more support.

Hypopressives

The technique has given hope to people who felt at a loss after being diagnosed with prolapse. Many people have been told they can never run or lift again so have avoided these activities or stopped doing them out of fear of making things worse. Hypopressive low pressure fitness has been a game changer for me and many of my clients. Bladder prolapse is typically the first to respond and perhaps the easiest to address due to the attachment of the urachus which is a midline tubular structure that joins the apex of the bladder and the umbilicus. During an apnea, the vacuum effect draws the belly button up, which in turn draws the bladder up as well. The position of the uterus resting above the bladder is therefore also pulled up to some degree. The rectum is influenced myofascially as well, but is much slower to respond and harder to reverse.

There are many anecdotal stories of people reversing early stage (stage 1–2) bladder and uterine prolapse and some have brought a stage 3 up a level to a stage 2. Many of my clients report that the day after a hypopressive session they feel less symptomatic even when they are first learning the technique. Change is very motivating.

There are more and more trainers and physios becoming certified in the technique and it is ideal if you can work one-on-one with someone, but there are some online programmes that can help you learn the technique if there is no trainer in your area. You can visit lowpressurefitness.com or www.ukhypopressives.com/ to search for a trainer in your area.

APPENDIX 2: THE CORE COLLABORATORS

If you'd like a bit more background on the workings of the body, and how strengthening your pelvic floor is about SO MUCH MORE than just the pelvic floor working in isolation, here is a break down of the other players on the team.

Nothing works in isolation in our bodies. Like an orchestra where each plays an integral part in creating the music. We are a masterfully interconnected group of systems that allow us to eat, move, breathe, poo and procreate. The Core Four work synergistically, but not alone. The psoas, piriformis, quadratus lumborum, glutes, adductors and obturator internus also attach to or influence the pelvis and need to be considered as well.

The psoas
The psoas muscles begin at your 12th rib and attach on each of the lumbar vertebrae, then run through and over the front of the pelvis to attach on the upper femur. Because of the attachment points on the ribs and lumbar vertebrae, it greatly influences the spine and the pelvis. The psoas is generally considered a hip flexor, and also a spinal stabilizer. It's also involved in external rotation of the hip.

When the upper portion is tight, it can pull the spine forward and down, which can contribute to rib flaring or rib thrusting. When the psoas is tight in the lumbar region, it can pull the lumbar vertebrae forward and down and can contribute to swayback posture. If the lower portion is tight, it can pull the femur forward in the hip socket, which can tip the pelvis posteriorly. The psoas are typically short and tight in people who sit a lot and it is also through to be a muscle that holds on to fear and emotion. Exercises to lengthen the psoas and release tension can offer tremendous relief for back pain in many people.

The piriformis
The piriformis is considered a pelvic wall muscle. It arises from the anterior sacrum and inserts into the greater trochanter (leg bone). It plays a role in stabilizing the SI joint together with the psoas. A tight piriformis is often blamed for sciatica.

The quadratus lumborum
The quadratus lumborum (QL) attaches the pelvis to the rib cage and lies very close to the psoas as well as the iliacus muscles that line the inside of the pelvis. The QL is considered a postural muscle that stabilizes the diaphragm on inspiration. There's also been a relationship shown between kyphosis (a rounded upper back) in sitting and a tight QL.

The glutes
The glute muscles attach to the sacrum and posterior pelvis as well as the femur (thigh bone). They help contribute to lateral hip control and can help keep the sacrum in its optimal position. The glutes help tension the thoracolumbar fascia and also work in coordination with the pelvic floor which makes them a very important muscle group for diastasis recti and pelvic floor challenges.

The adductors

The adductors, or inner thighs, attach at the pubic joint of the pelvis and facilitate activation of the pelvic floor muscles. It is common for some people to overuse this muscle group when stability in the pelvis is lacking. We *don't* want this muscle to be squeezing when we're engaging our pelvic floor.

The obturator internus

The obturator internus (OI) is considered a pelvic wall muscle and originates on the inner surface of the pelvis just below and to the side of the pubic joint. It attaches to the top of the femur (the greater trochanter). The OI shares fascial attachments with the pelvic floor muscles and strengthening the OI can play a role in improving or optimizing pelvic floor function.

APPENDIX 3: PESSARIES

Speak to your pelvic health physio about choosing the right pessary for you. In the UK there is less choice than in the States, so it is hard to be prescriptive here. Ask what there is available to you and persist until you find one that feels right for you.

With regards to which pessary is best for each prolapse it really does depend on the individual. For a guide, below is a summary of the most common pessaries and the type of prolapse they are most *often* used for so you at least have a starting point. You may need to try a few before finding the right form and fit for your body.

Cystocele (bladder prolapse)

- Shaatz
- Hodge
- Gehrung with or without knob
- Oval
- Marland
- Dish with support
- Incostress

Uterine prolapse

- Ring
- Donut
- Gelhorn
- Cube
- Inflatable
- Gehrung with or without knob
- Marland
- Shaatz

Rectocele

- Cube
- Gehrung
- Marland
- Inflatable

TIPS FROM THE GLOBAL PELVIC HEALTH VILLAGE

–

WHAT PELVIC EXPERTS SAY

Studies show it may take years, or even decades for some problems such as incontinence and chronic pain to show up after childbirth.

Once postpartum, always postpartum.

MARIANNE RYAN, PT
NEW YORK, NY USA
WWW.BABYBODBOOK.COM

As a physical therapist and yoga therapist, it has been extremely valuable to combine physical therapy and yoga when addressing a variety of pelvic health issues. I have found that focused meditations such as "body scanning" and "pelvic diaphragmatic breath awareness"' have been instrumental in creating a higher awareness of the pelvic floor, which is the first step prior to releasing, engaging or controlling the pelvic floor muscles .

One of the best pelvic health tips I recommend to men and women is to practice what I call the "Toilet Meditation". There are a few specific parts to the meditation; but in summary, it is simply being completely present and aware when performing your toilet duties! As you sit, scan the entire body and notice any areas of tension or physical sensations. Try to stay present in your body and aware of your breath, observing any thoughts that take you away from the present moment.

Focus on observing the natural rhythm of both the respiratory and the pelvic diaphragms as you breathe, releasing the pelvic floor and taking your time. We often rush when we urinate, and may not always fully empty our bladders. This can potentially result in a cascade of unwanted issues, or exacerbate existing issues such as persistent pelvic pain dysfunctions, over active bladder or incontinence, to name a few.

Part of optimal pelvic floor health starts with awareness, breathing, and ability to release the pelvic floor.

SHELLY PROSKO, PT
SYLVAN LAKE, AB CANADA
WWW. PHYSIOYOGA.CA

During attempted vaginal penetration, if it feels as if your partner is "hitting a wall", whether it be difficulty inserting a penis, dildo, finger, or sex toy, stop! Pelvic floor disorders can make vaginal penetration difficult or impossible, and persevering through the pain will worsen the situation.

DR LORI BROTTO
VANCOUVER, BC CANADA
WWW.BROTTOLAB.COM

I wish everyone knew that they should not go to the bathroom "just in case."

This typically leads to increased urinary urge and frequency during the day and can also cause one to have to wake up in the middle of the night to go. I give my patients a challenge – try to avoid going to the bathroom just in case. Rather wait at least 2–4 hours and within 2 weeks, there should be a change noticed. This can require baby steps at first, but it can be life changing.

TRACY SHER, PT
ORLANDO, FL USA
WWW.SHERPELVIC.COM
WWW.PELVICGURU.COM

ALL WORK IS NOT EQUAL. THE ACTIVITY YOU ARE DOING DICTATES THE WORK YOUR FLOOR HAS TO DO i.e.: putting on your socks does not require the same pelvic floor activation that moving a fridge does. Once your PF is automated, or at least something you don't have to think of as often, you can ramp up the work when needed (moving the fridge) and hopefully breathe and move with ease and trusting your PF is firing just as much as it needs to.

LAURA APPS, PT
AJAX, ON CANADA
WWW.WOMENSHEALTHPHYSIO.CA

One of the earliest signs of vulvar or vaginal cancer can be skin changes. Most women are aware of the benefits of doing regular sBe's (self-breast exams) but few (unfortunately) are doing regular vulvar self-exams.

Position yourself comfortably, propped up in bed. Make sure your hands are clean. Don't use any creams or lotions, as this may interfere with your ability to detect any changes. Holding a mirror in one hand and use your other hand to separate the labia and look at your vulva. Check the clitoris and the surrounding area.

Then move down to the vaginal opening. Check the small folds of skin to the left and right. Now move down to the area around the anal opening because vulvar disease can spread to here. If you notice:

- Any lumps, bumps or skin changes
- Itching
- Pain
- Burning sensation, especially after urinating
- Any unusual discharge
- That you bleed after sex
- That you bleed between periods OR after menopause make an appointment to see your doctor.

MICHELLE LYONS, PT
FORE, WESTMEATH, IRELAND
WWW.CELEBRATEMULIEBRITY.COM

If we were animals walking on all fours, prolapse wouldn't be an issue because our organs would have great support from the pubic bone and muscular wall of the abdomen. But since we walk upright, we have the effect of gravity weighing down on our organs which rely on strong pelvic floors to support them from beneath. There are little things you can do throughout the day to improve their support.

Sitting and standing in an upright posture with your pelvis titled forward and buttocks lifted slightly helps keep the organs nicely supported by the pubic bone rather than being positioned over the vaginal opening. Over the long haul, this can make a big difference to how much downwards pull gravity has on your organs.

— MUNIRA HUDANI, PT
TORONTO, ON CANADA
WWW.MUNIRAHUDANIPT.COM

There's no shame in finding out you are incontinent, the shame comes when you don't do anything about it but before buying products and gadgets, blind off the net, see a women's health physio for proper advice and help first. Your pelvic floor needs proper training. BEST TO SEEK TRAINING FROM THE PROFESSIONALS i.e. pelvic health physios, they know what they are doing and teach you how to best train yourself.

GAYNOR MORGAN
SOUTH WALES, UK
WWW.INCOSTRESS.COM

Learning to use your core correctly is not just for while you're "doing your exercises". Those few minutes of focus each day are great for re-connecting with your body and your muscles, but the time when you really need to look after your core, is the everyday stuff, when you have a child, heavy bags or the laundry to pick up!

WENDY POWELL
CORNWALL, UK
WWW. MUTUSYSTEM.COM

The pelvic floor muscle is my favourite group of muscles in the body! Take a moment and appreciate what a typical day in the life of this muscle might entail.

The amazing pelvic floor is silently working all day to protect us and we are usually oblivious to its critical contributions. Day and night it must contract and relax immediately, properly and efficiently to react to every pressure change in our body, from subtle to large. This could be as little as during a hiccup or when standing up from sitting, to protecting us when we need to lift something heavy, or keeping us safe during a 10 km run.

The pelvic floor muscles work to support us in healthy biomechanical postures and seamlessly transferring forces through the pelvis from our legs and trunk every time we move. These muscles are always "on the job", ensuring we don't accidentally pee or pass gas when we laugh or sneeze and ensuring we have a good and complete void and bowel movement when we decide the time is right. These muscles assist our diaphragm in respiration so they literally work with every breath we take!

And then, after working all day long, these wonderful muscles gives us the fulfilling orgasm we deserve to complete a perfect day.

DR. KELLY BERZUK
WINNIPEG, MB CANADA
WWW.NOVA- PHYSIO.COM

The pelvic floor and core both have a role in: STABILITY - BALANCE - DIGESTION - ORGAN SUPPORT - RESPIRATION - MOBILITY ELIMINATION - REPRODUCTION - EMOTION

Typically, we think pelvic floor/ core issues are present when we see symptoms like incontinence, pelvic organ prolapse, low sex drive or poor sexual response or pain in the pelvis. However, we also know that the following less known symptoms are also indicative of poor pelvic/core function:

- Poor balance or physical performance
- Irritable bowel, poor digestion, constipation
- Pain in back, hips, shoulders, the jaw
- Poor posture or misalignment, fatigue
- Mood disorders

If unaddressed, any one of these problems can lead to other wider psychological issues such as social isolation, relationship and intimacy issues, poor self-esteem and a decrease in physical activity.

We need to understand that our pelvic floor and our core are complicated and require so much more than kegels! To broaden our perspective – the pelvic floor, respiratory diaphragm, deep abdominals and the back muscles act like instruments in an orchestra.

They all need to do their part and play together to create beautiful and safe movement music. Of course we can't forget about the conductor of this orchestra, the brain! The brain coordinates this complex movement music through many feedback loops involving such things as hormones, nutrition, the nerves, emotions, somatic receptors and more.

We are so much more than muscles and bones. The key is to create an environment of availability within each of our bodies to allow the all of the systems to work together.

See a Certified Pelvic Health Physiotherapist to learn about how you can play beautiful music within your body and orchestrate beautiful movement!

CHERYL LEIA, PT
NORTH VANCOUVER, BC CANADA
WWW. PHYSIOTIQUES.COM

When doing pelvic floor exercises, make sure that once you have "got" the connection to the muscles, you start integrating them into core exercises and functional activity. It is not useful if the only time you can activate the muscles is flat on your back. I say that the pelvic floor is part of a "neighbourhood" of muscles and to be successful at pelvic floor strengthening, you need to integrate these muscles back into the neighbourhood so that they can be used functionally.

KATHLEEN SHORTT, PT
TORONTO, ON CANADA
WWW.INBALANCEPHYSIO.CA

Choose a fitness style that blesses and benefits your pelvic floor. If your workout is wrecking your pelvic floor and not restoring, it's time to step back and reassess your program and goals. Definition isn't worth dysfunction. If your exercise regimen is increasing your incontinence issues or widening your diastasis recti, then it's too much for your body in your present state, and it's time to seek one-on-one rehab with a specialist and switch to restorative exercises. And this frustrating time when you need to slow down to move ahead again? Yeah, it's just a season, friend. Trust that if you give your body what it needs right now, it will give you what you need later. Honour your body's limits today, and your body will honor you by expanding those limits tomorrow. This isn't forever. You will get stronger again. But right now you need to put yourself back together with gentle movements and wholesome foods. And I believe you will look back on restful seasons in your life with fondness once you learn to embrace them.

BETHANY LEARN
VANCOUVER, WA USA
WWW.FIT2B.US

While we live in a busy world and rushing seems to be a daily sport, please resist the temptation to force or push pee out.

When doing so, you can bulge your pelvic floor outwards which does not help to maintain good muscle tone. Instead sit down, relax your sphincter and let gravity do its thing. You may not save time but you could reduce your pelvic floor stress.

TRISH BRUNELLE BHSC, PT
BARRIE, ON CANADA
WWW.GETMOVINGPHYSIO.COM

Observe your perineal area with a mirror every few months or so. Not only can you spot something that looks out of the ordinary, you can also gain valuable perspective and connection with your vulva: IT IS NOT A FORBIDDEN ZONE! Men get to see their parts up front and centre. We just have to go a little out of our way to look at ours. And while you are down there smile and do a kegel ... it might just wink back .

GAYLE HULME, PT
CALGARY, AB CANADA
WWW.LAKEVIEWPHYSIO.CA

Women around the world suffer in silence with symptoms they don't understand. Stigma has veiled pelvic organ prolapse (POP) in silence for nearly 4000 years, but as women navigating this extremely common condition come together to talk out loud about the impact to their quality of life, we will lift the veil, establish POP awareness, and generate the next big shift in women's health directives.

Pelvic organ prolapse is without a doubt the biggest secret in women's health. Women with POP are hungry for hope. We move forward side by side.

SHERRIE PALM
FOUNDER/EXECUTIVE DIRECTOR, ASSOCIATION
FOR PELVIC ORGAN PROLAPSE SUPPORT
WWW.PELVICORGANPROLAPSESUPPORT.ORG
WWW.SHERRIEPALM.COM

Over the years working as a physio, I've learned that sometimes the most obvious thing is the most overlooked. We often jump right into treating one thing or another, but in the words of that famous song from that famous musical, "Let's start at the very beginning," and what is the very beginning?

Awareness.

I'm talking about the ability of you and me to tune in, feel, perceive, and sense — to sense where we are in space, to feel the subtleties of our daily postures and positions, to appreciate the nuances in our movements, and to notice the connections between seemingly unrelated body parts.

Awareness is the starting point in pelvic health physiotherapy because it is essential to everything that we subsequently do. Developing that sense of mind-body awareness means that you can really know, reconnect to, and hopefully appreciate the amazing system that is your body. It allows you to take control over your pain or dysfunction, instead of letting it control you. It means that you can begin to make changes and improvements to your health on the micro and macro levels. It ultimately helps to rewire and retrain your brain, neural pathways, and motor patterns. When you begin to develop this perceptual ability, it really is amazing how much more you can feel and the overall impact on your pelvic health. Feeling is the key to healing.

So before starting anything else, before breathing, or visualizations, or kegels, or any other exercise, I usually say something that goes a little bit like this: "Close your eyes, quiet your mind, concentrate, and feel ..."

IBUKUN AFOLABI, PT
LONDON, ON, CANADA
WWW.THEMAMASPHYSIO.COM

Your path to healing lies within you.

You have to be strong and have courage in the face of adversity. Listen to the messages from your body, have a strong intention to awaken the healer within you. Always remember you are more than just the story of your pain, and that true healing must occur on all aspects of your being, emotional, physical, and spiritual.

ISA HERRERA, MSPT, CSCS
NEW YORK, NY USA
WWW.RENEWPT.COM

The action of a pelvic floor contraction is close and lift.

Most anatomical diagrams show everything sitting up with the organs lined up like soldiers, when in reality the orientation of your pelvic floor and organs is forwards. If you stand up and feel where your hip bone is you will feel that your pelvis is tilted forwards, and if you put a finger on your anus think about where it will "lift" to – towards your pubic bone.

FIONA ROGERS, PT
SIPPY DOWNS, QUEENSLAND AUSTRALIA
WWW.PELVICFLOOREXERCISE.COM.AU

RESOURCES AND USEFUL ORGANIZATIONS

Pelvic Floor Exercises and Equipment

Elvie is an award-winning pelvic floor trainer that uses biofeedback to help you track your progress
www.elvie.com

Squeezy is an award-winning app endorsed by the NHS
www.squeezyapp.com

www.epi-no.com

www.intimaterose.com

www.kegelbell.com

Pregnancy, Birth and Motherhood

The Ab Wrap
Sold through Bellies Inc.

The American College of Obstetricians and Gynaecology
Website offers useful information for pelvic floor concerns relating to childbirth
www.acog.org

The MASIC Foundation – Mothers with Anal Sphincter Injuries in Childbirth
Raising awareness to reduce the incidence of birth injuries, as well as helping new mothers who may be suffering in silence from pelvic floor trauma.
www.masic.org.uk

Mumsnet – advice and support from other parents www.mumsnet.com
www.mumsnet.com

Pelvic, Obstetric and Gynaecological Physiotherapy (POGP)
www.pogp.csp.org.uk

Pessaries
C&G Medicare is a pessary provider that has a fantastic shop with great education and support.

The Royal College of Midwives
www.rcm.org.uk

The Royal College of Obstetricians and Gynaecologists
Provides resources for women regarding pelvic floor health and childbirth.
www.rcog.org.uk

Return to Running Guidelines
https://www.absolute.physio/wp-content/uploads/2019/09/returning-to-running-postnatal-guidelines.pdf
Tom Goom, Grainne Donnelly and Emma Brockwell

Menopause

International Menopause Society
www.imsociety.org

Menopause Chicks
www.menopausechicks.com
North American Menopause Society
www.menopause.org

Women's Health Concern
www.womens-health-concern.org

Sex

The British Society for the Study of Vulval Diseases
https://bssvd.org

The Vulval Pain Society
www.vulvalpainsociety.org

Incontinence and Bowel issues

Bowel Disorders: The Rome Criterior for constipation
https://theromefoundation.org/wp-content/uploads/bowel-disorders.pdf\

Bowel Disease Research Foundation
www.bdrf.org.uk

The Bladder and Bowel Community
www.bladderandbowel.org

Squatty Potty
www.squattypotty.com

The "Go Better" stool
www.stressnomore.co.uk

The Great British Toilet Map
The UK's database of accessible public toilets
www.toiletmap.org.uk

The International Continence Society
www.ics.org

Useful Websites

www.vaginacoach.com

www.coreconfidenceeducation.com

https://pelvicguru.com/directory/

https://estrogenmatters.com/

www.kegelreleasecurve.com

www.pelvicorganprolapsesupport.org/sherrie-palm

https://joylux.com/ (vsculpt)

www.incostress.co.uk/shop/ (pessaries)

Pelvic Organ Prolapse Support (APOPS)

Pelvic Roar www.pelvicroar.org

Books

Bowman, Katy *Move Your DNA*

Bluming, Avrum and Carol Tavris *Estrogen Matters*

Brett, Luce, *PMSL: Or How I Literally Pissed Myself Laughing and Survived the Last Taboo to Tell the Tale*

Kalinik, Eve, *Be Good To Your Gut*

Ou, Heng, *The First Forty Days*

ENDNOTES

Chapter 2

1 Chmielewska D, Stania M, Słomka K, et al. Static postural stability in women with stress urinary incontinence: effects of vision and bladder filling. *Neurourol Urodyn.* 2017;36(8):2019–2027. doi:10.1002/nau.23222

2 Melville JL, Katon W, Delaney K, Newton K. Urinary incontinence in US women: a population-based study. *Arch Intern Med.* 2005;165(5):537–542. doi:10.1001/archinte.165.5.537

3 Nygaard IE, Thompson FL, Svengalis SL, Albright JP. Urinary incontinence in elite nulliparous athletes [published correction appears in *Obstet Gynecol* 1994 Sep;84(3):342]. *Obstet Gynecol.* 1994;84(2):183–187.

4 Shaw JM, Hamad NM, Coleman TJ, et al. Intra-abdominal pressures during activity in women using an intra-vaginal pressure transducer. *J Sports Sci.* 2014;32(12):1176–1185. doi:10.1080/02640414.2014.889845

5 O'Dell KK, Morse AN, Crawford SL, Howard A. Vaginal pressure during lifting, floor exercises, jogging, and use of hydraulic exercise machines. *Int Urogynecol J Pelvic Floor Dysfunct.* 2007;18(12):1481–1489. doi:10.1007/s00192-007-0387-8

6 Hagen S, Stark D. Conservative prevention and management of pelvic organ prolapse in women.

Cochrane Database Syst Rev. 2011;(12):CD003882. doi:10.1002/14651858.CD003882.pub4

7   Whiteside JL, Weber AM, Meyn LA, Walters MD. Risk factors for prolapse recurrence after vaginal repair. *Am J Obstet Gynecol.* 2004;191(5):1533–1538. doi:10.1016/j.ajog.2004.06.109

8   Salvatore S, Siesto G, Serati, M. Risk factors for recurrence of genital prolapse. *Current Opinion in Obstetrics and Gynecology.* October 2010– Volume 22 – Issue 5 – p 420–424. doi: 10.1097/GCO.0b013e32833e4974

9   Wu WH, Meijer OG, Uegaki K, et al. Pregnancy-related pelvic girdle pain (PPP), I: Terminology, clinical presentation, and prevalence. *Eur Spine J.* 2004;13(7):575–589. doi:10.1007/s00586-003-0615-y

10 Signorello LB, Harlow BL, Chekos AK, Repke JT. Postpartum sexual functioning and its relationship to perineal trauma: a retrospective cohort study of primiparous women. *Am J Obstet Gynecol.* 2001;184(5):881–890. doi:10.1067/mob.2001.113855

11 Schwarzer AC, Aprill CN, Bogduk N. The sacroiliac joint in chronic low back pain. *Spine (Phila Pa 1976).* 1995;20(1):31–37. doi:10.1097/00007632-199501000-00007

12 Eliasson K, Elfving B, Nordgren B, Mattsson E. Urinary incontinence in women with low back pain. *Man Ther.* 2008;13(3):206–212. doi:10.1016/j.math.2006.12.006

13 Pool-Goudzwaard AL, Slieker ten Hove MC, Vierhout ME, et al. Relations between pregnancy-related low back pain, pelvic floor activity and pelvic floor dysfunction. *Int Urogynecol J Pelvic Floor Dysfunct.* 2005;16(6):468–474. doi:10.1007/s00192-005-1292-7

14 Dufour S, Vandyken B, Forget MJ, Vandyken C. Association between lumbopelvic pain and pelvic floor dysfunction in women: a cross sectional study. *Musculoskelet Sci Pract.* 2018;34:47–53. doi:10.1016/j.msksp.2017.12.001

Chapter 3

1   Lin F, Parthasarathy S, Taylor SJ, Pucci D, Hendrix RW, Makhsous M. Effect of different sitting postures on lung capacity, expiratory flow, and lumbar lordosis. *Arch Phys Med Rehabil.* 2006;87(4):504–509. doi:10.1016/j.apmr.2005.11.031

2   Mattox TF, Lucente V, McIntyre P, Miklos JR, Tomezsko J. Abnormal spinal curvature and its relationship to pelvic organ prolapse. *Am J Obstet Gynecol.* 2000;183(6):1381–1384. doi:10.1067/mob.2000.111489

3   Lee K. Activation of pelvic floor muscle during ankle posture change on the basis of a three-dimensional motion analysis system. *Med Sci Monit.* 2018;24:7223–7230. doi:10.12659/MSM.912689

4   Thompson JA, O'Sullivan PB, Briffa NK, Neumann P. Differences in muscle activation patterns during pelvic floor muscle contraction and Valsalva maneuver. *Neurourol Urodyn.* 2006;25(2):148–155. doi:10.1002/nau.20203

5   Hextall A, Bidmead J, Cardozo L, Hooper R. The impact of the menstrual cycle on urinary symptoms and the results of urodynamic investigation. *BJOG.* 2001 Nov;108(11):1193–1196. https://www.ncbi.nlm.nih.gov/pmc/articles/PMC4247226/

6   De Graaff AA, D'Hooghe TM, Dunselman GA, et al. The significant effect of endometriosis on physical, mental and social wellbeing: results from an international cross-sectional survey. *Hum Reprod.* 2013;28(10):2677–2685. doi:10.1093/humrep/det284

7   Yeung P Jr, Sinervo K, Winer W, Albee RB Jr. Complete laparoscopic excision of endometriosis in teenagers: is postoperative hormonal suppression necessary? *Fertil Steril.* 2011;95(6):1909–1912.e1. doi:10.1016/j.fertnstert.2011.02.037

8   Vannuccini S, Petraglia F. Recent advances in understanding and managing adenomyosis. *F1000Research*

2019, 8(F1000 Faculty Rev):283. doi:10.12688/
f1000research.17242.1

9   National Centre for Health Statistics. Key statistics from
the National Survey of Family Growth: Hysterectomy.
https://www.cdc.gov/nchs/nsfg/key_statistics/h.
htm#hysterectomy

10 McLennan MT, Harris JK, Kariuki B, Meyer S. Family
history as a risk factor for pelvic organ prolapse. *Int
Urogynecol J Pelvic Floor Dysfunct*. 2008;19(8):1063–1069.
doi:10.1007/s00192-008-0591-1

11 Family history increases the risk of incontinence. *BMJ*.
2004;329(7471):0-b. doi: 10.1136/bmj.329.7471.0-b

12 Young N, Atan IK, Rojas RG, Dietz HP. Obesity: how
much does it matter for female pelvic organ prolapse?.
Int Urogynecol J. 2018;29(8):1129–1134. doi:10.1007/
s00192-017-3455-8

13 Subak LL, King WC, Belle SH, et al. Urinary incontinence
before and after bariatric surgery. *JAMA Intern Med*. 2015
Aug;175(8):1378–1387.

14 Myers DL, Sung VW, Richter HE, Creasman J, Subak
LL. Prolapse symptoms in overweight and obese women
before and after weight loss. *Female Pelvic Med Reconstr
Surg*. 2012 Jan–Feb; 18(1):55–59. doi:10.1097/
SPV.0b013e31824171f9

15 Braekken IH, Majida M, Ellström Engh M, Holme IM,
Bø K. Pelvic floor function is independently associated
with pelvic organ prolapse. *BJOG*. 2009;116(13):1706–
1714. doi:10.1111/j.1471-0528.2009.02379.x

16 Nygaard IE, Shaw JM. Physical activity and the pelvic
floor. *Am J Obstet Gynecol*. 2016;214(2):164–171.
doi:10.1016/j.ajog.2015.08.067

17 Forner LB, Beckman EM, Smith MD. Symptoms of
pelvic organ prolapse in women who lift heavy weights
for exercise: a cross-sectional survey. *Int Urogynecol J*.
2020;31(8):1551–1558. doi:10.1007/s00192-019-
04163-w

18 Shaw JM, Nygaard IE. Role of chronic exercise on pelvic floor support and function. *Curr Opin Urol.* 2017;27(3):257–261. doi:10.1097/ MOU.0000000000000390

19 Mitchell I, Evans L, Rees T, Hardy L. Stressors, social support, and tests of the buffering hypothesis: effects on psychological responses of injured athletes. *Br J Health Psychol.* 2014;19(3):486–508. doi:10.1111/bjhp.12046

20 Fischer MJ, Riedlinger K, Gutenbrunner C, Bernateck M. Influence of the temporomandibular joint on range of motion of the hip joint in patients with complex regional pain syndrome. *J Manipulative Physiol Ther.* 2009;32(5):364–371. doi:10.1016/j.jmpt.2009.04.003

Chapter 4

1 Mørkved S, Bø K, Schei B, Salvesen KA. Pelvic floor muscle training during pregnancy to prevent urinary incontinence: a single-blind randomized controlled trial. *Obstet Gynecol.* 2003;101(2):313–319. doi:10.1016/s0029-7844(02)02711-4

2 Viktrup L, Lose G. Lower urinary tract symptoms 5 years after the first delivery. *Int Urogynecol J Pelvic Floor Dysfunct.* 2000;11(6):336–340. doi:10.1007/ s001920070002

3 Glazener CM, Herbison GP, MacArthur C, Grant A, Wilson PD. Randomised controlled trial of conservative management of postnatal urinary and faecal incontinence: six year follow up. *BMJ.* 2005;330(7487):337. doi:10.1136/bmj.38320.613461.82

4 Williams A, Herron-Marx S, Knibb R. The prevalence of enduring postnatal perineal morbidity and its relationship to type of birth and birth risk factors. *J Clin Nurs.* 2007;16(3):549–561. doi:10.1111/j.1365-2702.2006.01593.x

5   Fritel X, Fauconnier A. Letter to the editor. Re: First
    vaginal delivery at an older age: does it carry an extra risk
    for the development of stress urinary incontinence? Groutz
    A, Helpman L, Gold R, Pauzner D, Lessing JB, Gordon D.
    2007. Neurourol Urodyn 26:779–782. *Neurourol Urodyn.*
    2009;28(4):365–366. doi:10.1002/nau.20608

6   Spitznagle TM, Leong FC, Van Dillen LR. Prevalence
    of diastasis recti abdominis in a urogynecological patient
    population. *Int Urogynecol J Pelvic Floor Dysfunct.*
    2007;18(3):321–328. doi:10.1007/s00192-006-0143-5

7   Mota P, Pascoal AG, Carita AI, Bø K. Normal width
    of the inter-recti distance in pregnant and postpartum
    primiparous women. *Musculoskelet Sci Pract.* 2018;35:34–
    37. doi:10.1016/j.msksp.2018.02.004

8   Lee D, Hodges PW. Behavior of the linea alba during a
    curl-up task in diastasis rectus abdominis: an observational
    study. *J Orthop Sports Phys Ther.* 2016;46(7):580–589.
    doi:10.2519/jospt.2016.6536

9   Frohlich J, Kettle C. Perineal care. *BMJ Clin Evid.* 2015
    Mar 10;2015:1401.

10 Villot A, Deffieux X, Demoulin G, Rivain AL, Trichot
    C, Thubert T. Prise en charge des périnées complets
    (déchirure périnéale stade 3 et 4) : revue de la littérature
    [Management of third and fourth degree perineal tears:
    a systematic review]. *J Gynecol Obstet Biol Reprod (Paris).*
    2015;44(9):802–811. doi:10.1016/j.jgyn.2015.06.005

11 Sundquist JC. Long-term outcome after obstetric
    injury: a retrospective study. *Acta Obstet Gynecol
    Scand.* 2012;91(6):715–718. doi:10.1111/j.1600-
    0412.2012.01398.x

12 Allen VM, Baskett TF, O'Connell CM, McKeen D, Allen,
    AC. Maternal and perinatal outcomes with increasing
    duration of the second stage of labor. *Obstetrics &
    Gynecology*: June 2009 – Volume 113 – Issue 6 – p 1248–
    1258. doi: 10.1097/AOG.0b013e3181a722d6

13 Ashton-Miller JA, Delancey JO. On the biomechanics
    of vaginal birth and common sequelae. *Annu Rev
    Biomed Eng.* 2009;11:163–176. doi:10.1146/annurev-
    bioeng-061008-124823

14 van Delft KW, Thakar R, Sultan AH, IntHout J,
    Kluivers KB. The natural history of levator avulsion one
    year following childbirth: a prospective study. *BJOG.*
    2015;122(9):1266–1273. doi:10.1111/1471-0528.13223

15 Dietz HP, Simpson JM. Levator trauma is associated
    with pelvic organ prolapse. *BJOG.* 2008;115(8):979–984.
    doi:10.1111/j.1471-0528.2008.01751.x

16 Swenson CW, DePorre JA, Haefner JK, Berger MB,
    Fenner DE. Postpartum depression screening and pelvic
    floor symptoms among women referred to a specialty
    postpartum perineal clinic. *Am J Obstet Gynecol.*
    2018 Mar;218(3):335.e1–335.e6. doi:10.1016/j.
    ajog.2017.11.604

Chapter 6

1   Crotty K, Bartram CI, Pitkin J, et al. Investigation
    of optimal cues to instruction for pelvic floor muscle
    contraction: a pilot study using 2D ultrasound imaging in
    pre-menopausal, nulliparous, continent women. *Neurourol
    Urodyn.* 2011;30(8):1620–1626. doi:10.1002/nau.21083

2   Hagen S, Stark D. Conservative prevention and
    management of pelvic organ prolapse in women.
    Cochrane Database Syst Rev. 2011;(12):CD003882.
    doi:10.1002/14651858.CD003882.pub4

3   Marques A, Stothers L, Macnab A. The status of pelvic
    floor muscle training for women. *Can Urol Assoc J.*
    2010;4(6):419–424. doi:10.5489/cuaj.10026

4   Bø K, Talseth T, Holme I. Single blind, randomised
    controlled trial of pelvic floor exercises, electrical
    stimulation, vaginal cones, and no treatment in

management of genuine stress incontinence in women. *BMJ*. 1999;318(7182):487–493. doi:10.1136/bmj.318.7182.487

5 Farzinmehr A, Moezy A, Koohpayehzadeh J, Kashanian M. A comparative study of whole body vibration training and pelvic floor muscle training on women's stress urinary incontinence: three-month follow-up. *J Family Reprod Health*. 2015;9(4):147–154.

INDEX

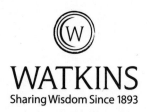

WATKINS
Sharing Wisdom Since 1893

The story of Watkins began in 1893, when scholar of esotericism John Watkins founded our bookshop, inspired by the lament of his friend and teacher Madame Blavatsky that there was nowhere in London to buy books on mysticism, occultism or metaphysics. That moment marked the birth of Watkins, soon to become the publisher of many of the leading lights of spiritual literature, including Carl Jung, Rudolf Steiner, Alice Bailey and Chögyam Trungpa.

Today, the passion at Watkins Publishing for vigorous questioning is still resolute. Our stimulating and groundbreaking list ranges from ancient traditions and complementary medicine to the latest ideas about personal development, holistic wellbeing and consciousness exploration. We remain at the cutting edge, committed to publishing books that change lives.

DISCOVER MORE AT:
www.watkinspublishing.com

Read our blog

Watch and listen to
our authors in action

Sign up to
our mailing list

We celebrate conscious, passionate, wise and happy living.
Be part of that community by visiting

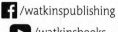 /watkinspublishing   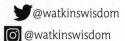 @watkinswisdom

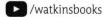 /watkinsbooks   @watkinswisdom